Springer
Tokyo
Berlin
Heidelberg
New York
Hong Kong
London
Milan
Paris

K. Okita (Ed.)

NASH and Nutritional Therapy

With 35 Figures, Including 5 in Color

Springer

Kiwamu Okita, M.D., Ph.D.
Professor and Chairman
Department of Gastroenterology and Hepatology
Yamaguchi University School of Medicine
1-1-1 Minami-Kogushi, Ube, Yamaguchi 755-8505, Japan

ISBN 4-431-21388-0 Springer-Verlag Tokyo Berlin Heidelberg New York

Library of Congress Control Number: 2004113088

This symposium was supported by funds from the Viral Hepatitis Research Foundation of Japan.

Printed on acid-free paper

Springer is a part of Springer Science+Business Media
springeronline.com

Typesetting: SNP Best-set Typesetter Ltd., Hong Kong
Printing and binding: Shinano Inc., Japan

Preface

Fatty liver disease including nonalcoholic steatohepatitis (NASH) involves the accumulation of triglycerides in hepatocytes with necrosis, inflammation, and often fibrosis with progression to cirrhosis. The two-hit model summarizes the important early metabolic events leading to hepatocellular necrosis in NASH. In these proceedings, we present various new findings and a review of NASH. The liver has an important role in nutritional homeostasis, and liver diseases lead to abnormalities in nutrient metabolism and to subsequent malnutrition, especially in patients with liver cirrhosis. Protein-energy malnutrition (PEM) is a common finding in cirrhotic patients; it may be present in 20% of patients with well-compensated disease and in more than 60% of patients with severe liver insufficiency. Therefore, special attention is required in the management of those patients; proper nutritional assessment and support for cirrhotic patients is essential. This volume also includes new findings on the nutritional aspects of the treatment of liver cirrhosis, which we hope will contribute to a better understanding of NASH and nutritional treatment.

We thank Otsuka Pharmaceutical Co. Ltd. for their continuing support.

Organizing Committee of the Yamaguchi Symposium on Liver Disease

Kiwamu Okita, M.D., Yamaguchi University, Ube
Masamichi Kojiro, M.D., Kurume University, Kurume
Masao Omata, M.D., The University of Tokyo, Tokyo
Norio Hayashi, M.D., Osaka University, Osaka
Takeshi Okanoue, M.D., Kyoto Prefectural University of Medicine, Kyoto

Secretary General

Isao Sakaida, M.D., Yamaguchi University, Ube

Table of Contents

List of Participants

Caldwell, Stephen H.	Division of Gastroenterology and Hepatology University of Virginia Health System Virginia, USA
Enzan, Hideaki	First Department of Pathology, Kochi Medical School Kochi, Japan
Hashimoto, Etsuko	Institute of Gastroenterology Tokyo Women's Medical University, Tokyo, Japan
Hayashi, Norio	Department of Molecular Therapeutics Osaka University Graduate School of Medicine Osaka, Japan
Hino, Keisuke	Department of Laboratory Sciences, Faculty of Health Sciences, Yamaguchi University School of Medicine Yamaguchi, Japan
Ichida, Takafumi	Third Department of Internal Medicine, Niigata University Niigata, Japan
Ikejima, Kenichi	Department of Gastroenterology Juntendo University School of Medicine, Tokyo, Japan
Kodama, Takahiro	Department of Internal Medicine/Gastroenterology Yamaguchi Central Hospital, Yamaguchi, Japan
Kojiro, Masamichi	First Department of Pathology Kurume University School of Medicine, Fukuoka, Japan
Nakanishi, Toshio	Department of Radiology, School of Medicine Hiroshima University, Hiroshima, Japan
Nishiguchi, Shuhei	Department of Hepatology, Graduate School of Medicine Osaka City University, Osaka, Japan
Okanoue, Takeshi	Third Department of Internal Medicine Kyoto Prefectural University of Medicine, Kyoto, Japan

Okita, Kiwamu	Department of Gastroenterology and Hepatology Yamaguchi University School of Medicine Yamaguchi, Japan
Omata, Masao	Department of Gastroenterology Graduate School of Medicine, The University of Tokyo Tokyo, Japan
Onishi, Saburo	Department of Internal Medicine, Kochi Medical School Kochi, Japan
Saibara, Toshiji	Department of Internal Medicine, Kochi Medical School Kochi, Japan
Sakaida, Isao	Department of Gastroenterology and Hepatology Yamaguchi University School of Medicine Yamaguchi, Japan
Sata, Michio	Second Department of Medicine Kurume University School of Medicine, Kurume, Japan
Tanikawa, Kyuichi	International Institute for Liver Research, Fukuoka, Japan
Terai, Shuji	Department of Gastroenterology and Hepatology Yamaguchi University School of Medicine Yamaguchi, Japan
Tokushige, Katsutoshi	Institute of Gastroenterology Tokyo Women's Medical University, Tokyo, Japan
Tsuchiya, Masako	Department of Gastroenterology and Hepatology Yamaguchi University School of Medicine Yamaguchi, Japan
Ueno, Takato	Research Center for Innovative Cancer Therapy Kurume University School of Medicine, Kurume, Japan
Yonezawa, Kazuyoshi	Biosignal Research Center, Kobe University, Kobe, Japan

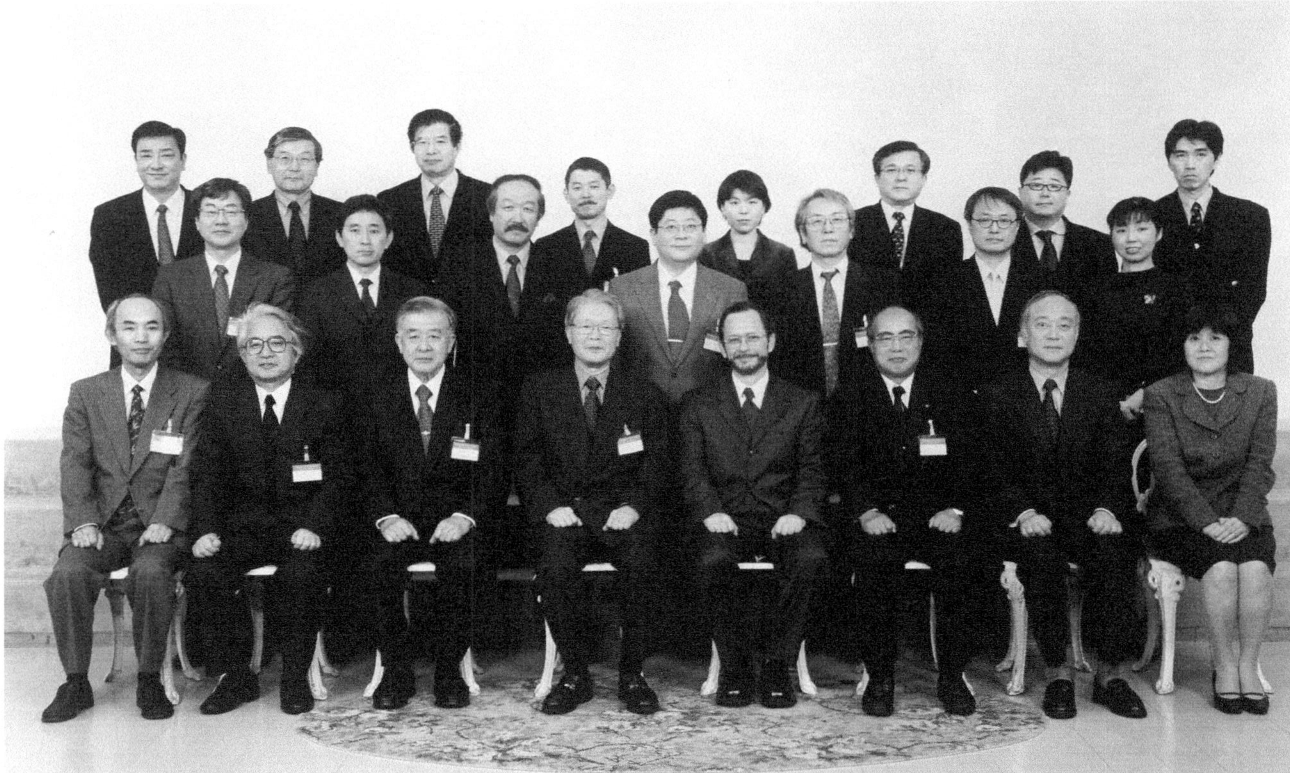

15th YAMAGUCHI SYMPOSIUM ON LIVER DISEASE
2003.12.6~7

Nonalcoholic Fatty Liver (NAFL): Overview

Stephen H. Caldwell[1], Abdullah Al-Osaimi[1], Charissa Chang[1], Christie Davis[1], Elizabeth E. Hespenheide[1], Lisa Krugner-Higby[2], Anita Impaglizzo Hylton[1], Julia C. Iezzoni[1], Tri H. Le[3], Robert K. Nakamoto[1], Jan Redick[1], and Theresa Peterson[4]

Summary. Nonalcoholic fatty liver (NAFL) or nonalcoholic fatty liver *disease* (NAFLD) as it is often called, is increasingly recognized as a common and potentially severe condition often associated with obesity, type 2 diabetes, and hyperlipidemia. The spectrum of disorders which fall under the term 'NAFL' include simple steatosis, steatosis with mild inflammation, and steatosis with inflammation and varying degrees of fibrosis. Most investigators reserve the term 'NASH' (nonalcoholic steatohepatitis) for those patients who have some degree of fibrosis, usually associated with increased numbers of ballooned hepatocytes. The prognosis varies, but it is now evident that a substantial portion of patients, especially those with NASH, will progress to cirrhosis with all of the attendant complications, and some may ultimately develop hepatocellular cancer. Well-developed cirrhosis may lose its fat content and appear as 'cryptogenic cirrhosis'. Lipid peroxidation of the excess oil in the liver appears to be the major pathogenic mechanism. The process appears to alter mitochondrial form and function. Initial treatment usually involves exercise and dietary modifications. Patients who fail this approach or who have more advanced conditions initially may be candidates for more aggressive measures, including drug therapy. Many agents have been reported in small series but all remain investigational.

Key words. Nonalcoholic fatty liver, Nonalcoholic steatohepatitis, Cryptogenic cirrhosis, Obesity, Type 2 diabetes

Introduction

The histologic findings in patients with NAFL vary widely in the degree of microscopic injury from none or minimal to cirrhosis. Although still somewhat controversial, the natural history and prognosis is variable between simple steatosis (sometimes referred to as 'pure' fatty liver), steatosis with inflammation, and steatosis with fibro-

[1] Division of Gastroenterology and Hepatology, Box 800708, University of Virginia Health System, Charlottesville, Virginia 22908-0708, USA
[2] The Research Animal Resources Center, University of Wisconsin-Madison, Madison, Wisconsin 53726-4089, USA
[3] Penn State Hershey Medical Center, 500 University Drive, Hershey, Pennsylvania 17033, USA
[4] Dalhousie University, Halifax, Nova Scotia B3H 4R2, Canada

sis. These forms of NAFL have been united into a classification system [1]. Predictive factors of more severe histology have also been determined and, to a lesser extent, the prevalence of NAFL types within different high-risk groups (obesity, diabetes, hyperlipidemia) has come into focus. Insulin resistance (IR) appears to be a common condition in NAFL, but it appears not to be uniformly present. Recently, Cotrim et al. [2] in Brazil have described NASH in petrochemical workers without an elevated index of IR. In addition, it seems likely that some forms of NAFL involve primary problems with lipoprotein metabolism, raising concerns about the potential toxicity of 'statin' drugs, which has been very little investigated. Thus, NAFL probably exists as a spectrum of disorders, although that seen with obesity and type 2 diabetes is the most common form.

Historical Perspective

The association between obesity and liver injury has been known since the 1800s [3, 4]. Several papers in the mid-1900s further reported a relationship between steatosis, progressive liver injury, and obesity [5]. Later, the association between intestinal bypass and progressive steatohepatitis further raised awareness of this disease [6]. However, even after the publication of several landmark papers in the 1980s (including that of Ludwig et al. [7], which provided the disease with its most common appellation 'NASH'), it became commonly taught that 'fatty liver' was a benign condition warranting little concern. While these misconceptions have largely given way to a much broader concept of fatty liver, there remains a good deal of lingering doubt about the overall prognosis and treatment of this condition.

Defining Terms in NAFL

In spite of recent progress, the nomenclature in NAFL has remained controversial and a consensus on working terminology has emerged largely by default [8]. Although the term 'NAFLD' is commonly used, we have elected to use the term 'NAFL' or 'nonalcoholic fatty liver' rather than 'NAFLD' or 'nonalcoholic fatty liver *disease*' since the disease portion of the latter term is variable and is not yet established for all of the forms of NAFL. We have reserved the term 'NASH' or 'nonalcoholic steatohepatitis' for more severe forms of NAFL (type 3–4), as described below.

The diagnosis of NAFL depends on the presence of an abnormal amount of fat in the liver. Prior studies demonstrated that the normal liver contains less than 5% fat by weight [9]. Since weight measurements are clinically impractical and most imaging modalities lack sensitivity (see below), fatty liver is most accurately diagnosed by light microscopy of biopsy specimens, although sampling error remains a potential problem. The cutoff level for significant steatosis has varied in the literature, but steatosis can be said to be present when the percentage of fat-laden hepatocytes exceeds a minimum of 5%–10% of the hepatocytes. The other major criterion implied in the term 'NAFL' is the issue of what constitutes 'nonalcoholic'. Levels defined as insignificant are also variable in the literature. Recently, some measure of agreement has been reached, allowing approximately 20 g per day (14 units per week) as a cutoff below which steatosis is 'nonalcoholic' [10].

'Presumptive' NAFL

A number of studies have utilized noninvasive studies to estimate the prevalence of steatosis in large populations wherein biopsy is impractical [11–13]. Most of these studies have utilized ultrasound examination of the liver for exclusion of other known diseases to make the diagnosis of 'presumed' NAFL. The noninvasive approach provides a practical means of assessing the prevalence of hepatic steatosis in a population under investigation, has utility in detecting other lesions, and finds clinical use as a screening for patients and potential living liver donors in the field of transplantation [14]. In addition, imaging can provide relevant information about body fat distribution by measuring indices of central adiposity [15]. However, no imaging technique has emerged which is capable of determining the presence or absence of histological injury.

This limitation was clearly demonstrated in a study by Saadeh et al. [16], in which 25 patients underwent biopsy (8 had mild NAFL and 17 had NASH), ultrasound, computed tomographic (CT) and magnetic resonance (MR) imaging. Steatosis of at least 33% was optimal for noninvasive imaging and values less than this were associated with substantial loss of sensitivity. None of the imaging modalities were useful in detecting histological features of NASH, such as balloon degeneration, Mallory hyaline, or fibrosis. Thus, although radiologic criteria exist to help guide the noninvasive diagnosis of NAFL [17–20], biopsy remains the gold standard for grading and staging of the disease. A possible exception is the use of MR spectroscopy, which has been shown to detect a physiological defect in ATP homeostasis in patients with NAFL [21]. Whether this modality or some combination of standard imaging and surrogate markers of histological injury will emerge as viable substitutes for biopsy remains to be seen (see below).

Histological Classification of NAFL

In their original study of 132 patients with NAFL, Matteoni et al. [1] grouped the biopsies into four groups: type 1 NAFL or simple steatosis, type 2 or steatosis with inflammation, and types 3 and 4, which were characterized by steatosis, inflammation and fibrosis, balloon cells, or Mallory bodies. There is a high degree of correlation between types 3 and 4, such that these should probably be put together as one group representing 'NASH' with several different stages of fibrosis. With a median follow-up of 8 years, cirrhosis developed much more commonly in the combined type 3–4 group (25%) than in the combined type 1–2 group (3%), and the crude liver-related mortality rate was also higher in the combined type 3–4 group. Other studies, by Hilden et al. [22] and Teli et al. [23], have supported the long-term stability of milder (types 1, 2) forms of NAFL. However, a transition from simple steatosis to a more aggressive form of NASH has been observed [24].

A close association between NAFL and cryptogenic cirrhosis has also been observed in a number of studies [25–28]. Similar to the histologic classification of NAFL, cryptogenic cirrhosis can be classified into several histological categories, including NASH with cirrhosis, cirrhosis with features of NASH (steatosis and glycogenated nuclei), and bland cirrhosis [29, 30].

These broad categories of NAFL and cryptogenic cirrhosis provide an important conceptual framework and attain a greater degree of importance by providing a basis on which to interpret clinical investigations and therapeutic trials through the use of a common set of terms. However, this system is based largely on only a few retrospective clinical studies and remains to be validated in additional prospective studies. The distinction between the various types of NAFL is not always clear-cut. In our experience, it is not uncommon to find a few scattered balloon cells (characteristic of type 3–4 NAFL) in a specimen with no fibrosis and only mild inflammation suggesting type 2 NAFL [31]. These and similar issues of precise histological definition are coming into sharper focus with increasing experience and refinements in the histological criteria [32, 33]. Of perhaps greatest importance is that investigators carefully define their terms in all reports to facilitate communications, whether or not they are using this classification scheme.

Epidemiology

NAFL is one of the most common of all liver disorders, but is among the most likely of liver disorders to be overlooked by primary care physicians [34]. The prevalence of all forms of NAFL has been estimated to be as high as 15%–20% of the adult population in the United States, Japan, and Italy [35]. Only about 20%–30% of these are thought to have the more severe form (NASH) but this is still quite a large fraction of the population in developed countries. Among obese people in western countries, about 60% have simple steatosis, 20%–25% have NASH, and 2%–3% have cirrhosis (see also below under 'Physical Findings') [36]. From the same publication, it was noted that at least 70% of type 2 diabetic patients have some form of fatty liver, and it has also been estimated that about 60% of hyperlipidemic patients have this disorder, although detailed histologic data have not, to our knowledge, been reported in these high-risk groups [37]. Among adults with NAFL, the metabolic syndrome (defined as three or more markers, including waist circumference, fasting hyperglycemia, elevated high-density lipoprotein [HDL], elevated triglycerides, or hypertension) is present in 88% of NASH patients and 54% of simple steatosis patients (see reference [30]). These figures are of even greater concern when considering the pediatric patient, where it is now estimated that more than 1%–2% of adolescents in the United States have some form of fatty liver (see reference [31]). The spectrum of histologic disease in the pediatric population can be severe [38].

History, Symptoms, and Physical Findings

As noted above, a history of obesity, diabetes, and/or hyperlipidemia is common, although not invariable. A family history of NASH or cryptogenic cirrhosis is frequent and warrants concern for a more progressive course [39, 40]. Other features of the 'metabolic syndrome' may be seen, such as hypertension, hyperuricemia, and the polycystic ovary syndrome [insulin resistance, diabetes, obesity, hirsutism, dysmenorrhea] [41–44]. Although widely associated with obesity (defined as body mass index [BMI] >30 kg/m^2 in people of primarily European or African descent) [45, 46], an increasing number of patients have been described with normal BMI, although most have central adiposity and latent or overt insulin resistance [47–50]. Waist circumference or the hip-waist ratio is probably the best anthropometric indicator of this sort of central obesity [51, 52], although use of special calipers to measure 'abdominal height' has been advocated. Changes in body composition due to aging and cirrhosis may mask a history of prior, severe, and longstanding obesity [53]. Thus, inquiry regarding past weight should be incorporated into the clinical evaluation.

Among obese individuals, the prevalence of NAFL and the expected frequency of different degrees of histologic injury can be estimated from past studies. Although much has to be conjectured because of the lack of common terminology, it can be approximated from a number of series that about 60% of obese individuals have relatively stable 'simple steatosis' or at most type 2 NAFL, while about 20%–25% have type 3–4 NAFL or frank NASH with fibrosis [54–58]. Only about 5% of such individuals have normal histology and about 5% have previously unrecognized cirrhosis. Whether or not these prevalence figures also apply to diabetic and hyperlipidemic patients is unknown, but warrants additional study. It is known that a substantial fraction of type 2 diabetic patients and hyperlipidemic patients have fatty infiltration by noninvasive testing [59, 60].

Common symptoms include fatigue and right upper quadrant pain, although the disorder even in the presence of cirrhosis may be silent. Associated conditions warrant consideration, including signs or symptoms of mitochondrialopathy-associated neuromuscular disease [61], gut motility [62, 63], lipodystrophy (fat atrophy) [64], lipomatosis [65], and Weber-Christian disease (panniculitis) [66]. A history of possible aggravating factors should be sought, including use of certain medications such as methotrexate, amiodarone, and tamoxifen [67–69], and solvent exposure [70]. Whether these variables aggravate a preexisting condition or cause a separate form of steatohepatitis (secondary NAFL) remains uncertain [71], but increasingly there appears to be a separate form of NAFL related to toxin exposure. Rarely, previously unrecognized NASH with silent cirrhosis may present as subacute liver failure [72]. More often these patients are discovered incidentally during some other evaluation [73], while up to 50% present initially with a major complication of cirrhosis such as ascites, variceal bleeding, or hepatocellular carcinoma [74].

Laboratory Findings in NAFL

Serum aminotransferase elevation, usually less than 1.5× normal [75], is perhaps the most common cause for patient referral [76–79]. The pattern of aspartate aminotransferase (AST) and alanine aminotransferase (ALT) elevation carries some additional prognostic significance (see below), but these values may be significantly altered in patients receiving medications for comorbidities such as diabetes and hyperlipidemia. NAFL is the most common cause of unexplained aminotransferase elevation in asymptomatic people [80]. Elevation appears to approximate the degree of inflammation, but less so for fibrosis. This is supported by early drug trials in NASH, which showed normalization of transaminases, reduced indices of inflammation, but no change in fibrosis with troglitazone therapy [81]. More recent studies using extended courses have, however, shown improvement in fibrosis scores (see below, under 'Current Therapy of NAFL: Antidiabetic and insulin sensitizing agents').

However, liver enzymes may be normal in spite of underlying disease [82]. This may represent the effects of 'burned-out' disease, the effects of drug therapy, as noted above, or an upward drift of the normal reference range over the past few years—a phenomenon, now being corrected, that is thought to have resulted from the unrecognized inclusion of NAFL and hepatitis C patients in the reference controls [83].

Other abnormalities include elevated iron indices, although usually without frank hemochromatosis [84–88], positive anti-nuclear antibody (ANA) in about 30% [89,90], elevation of serum IgA [91, 92], and mild abnormalities of alkaline phosphatase and gamma glutamyl transpeptidase (GGTP). Among patients with positive ANA, there does not appear to be any worsening of histology [93]. Slightly low ceruloplasmin levels without frank Wilson's disease are seen in about 10% of patients (unpublished observation). Markers of insulin resistance and sensitivity based on fasting insulin and glucose levels (Homeostasis Model Assessment [HOMA] and Quantitative insulin-sensitivity check index [QUICKI] tests) are increasingly being utilized in the clinical setting to assess these patients and their response to therapy [94]. These tests are essentially mathematical models referenced to the more elaborate and complicated hyperinsulinemic euglycemic clamp test. Markers of exercise tolerance and conditioning, such as the lactate threshold, will also likely find a role in clinically evaluating these patients but remain to be more thoroughly investigated. Recent studies have also begun to more carefully tease out the lipid profiles associated with NAFL [95].

The Role of Biopsy in the Diagnosis of NAFL

The biopsy remains the gold standard and serves to confirm the diagnosis and to stage the extent of injury in NASH. It is used early when the clinical evaluation is suspicious for more advanced disease or when there is a question of medication-induced injury. For those in whom the disease is not suspected to have significantly progressed, the biopsy is often deferred and a conservative course of exercise and diet is prescribed. Predictors of biopsy findings have been studied, although these should be regarded cautiously due to a high number of exceptions. Age more than 40–50 years, the degree of obesity, the degree of diabetes or insulin resistance, hypertriglyceridemia, hypertension, family history of NASH or cryptogenic cirrhosis, complete abstinence from ethanol, transaminase elevation, and an AST/ALT ratio of more than 1 are all predictive of more advanced histology on the initial biopsy [96–101]. Scores have been developed which include several parameters, but these remain to be validated. Whether these variables also predict the longterm course remains to be proven but seems likely. Female sex has not been a consistent predictor; however, the increasing prevalence of females with increasing fibrosis scores [102], and the preponderance of older females in most series of cryptogenic cirrhosis leave the issue unresolved. The discovery of unexpected cirrhosis at biopsy for NAFL is of obvious importance, as it casts the overall management of the obese, diabetic patient into a new light. Important considerations emerge if cirrhosis is discovered, such as avoidance of certain medications, and surveillance issues for varices or hepatocellular cancer.

Imaging studies (with the possible exception of MR spectroscopy) provide only limited information on the underlying pathophysiology. Markers of collagen and extracellular matrix metabolism have not been adequately studied, but may provide limited information [103]. Whether some combination of imaging such as contrast ultrasound [104] and collagen marker profiles [105] will emerge to replace some biopsies remains to be seen. Although biopsy is likely to remain the gold standard for establishing the diagnosis, advantages possessed by these noninvasive markers include a viable means of easily tracking treatment response and the potential avoidance of sampling error inherent with biopsy. The latter issue reflects the suspected existence of geographic variation within the NAFL—it is estimated that left and right lobe biopsies can vary in grade of activity in about 20% of patients [106]. Further propelling the field of noninvasive testing is the fact that liver biopsy is not without risk, and the lack of definitive therapy based on the results warrants caution in applying biopsy.

Fatal complications, usually hemorrhage, are estimated to occur in 1:10000 biopsies. Predicting this result is difficult, as the major problem is transgression of a vessel and bleeding risk correlates poorly to tests of coagulation [107]. Ultrasound guidance does not alter the risk of bleeding, which depends to a greater extent on the needle type (increased with larger needles and the cutting style) and the number of passes made [108]. However, the use of narrower gauge needles results in substantially less specimen and may compromise interpretation of the biopsy. Pain requiring intravenous analgesia occurs in 30%–50% of patients regardless of the use of ultrasound guidance [109], while more severe pain occurs in 1%–5% [110]. The body habitus of the patients most often afflicted with NAFL poses additional problems. While those with more central adiposity generally pose no significant problems for a percutaneous biopsy, those with more peripheral adipose tissue may require ultrasound guidance.

Prognosis: General

Although it is one of the most common of all liver disorders [111, 112], the natural history of NAFL remains a subject of active study. A substantial fraction of these patients will ultimately develop severe liver injury, presenting with new-onset ascites or variceal bleeding many years after the diagnosis of 'fatty liver'. Furthermore, it has become common to see older patients with 'cryptogenic cirrhosis' in the setting of prior known fatty liver, longstanding obesity, and type 2 diabetes. Advanced liver disease may become the dominant clinical problem in these patients, overtaking diabetes-related vascular disease. Not uncommonly, these patients eventually develop hepatocellular cancer.

The Prognosis of NAFL Based on Initial Histologic Classification

As mentioned earlier, a prognosis-related classification of NAFL has been proposed, although it remains to be validated in additional studies [113]. Some additional discussion of this work is warranted. Matteoni et al. [1] ascertained 132 patients with long-term follow-up and whose baseline biopsy, performed between 1979 and 1987, revealed NAFL. The biopsies were grouped into classes as follows: type 1 NAFL or simple steatosis, type 2 or steatosis with inflammation, and types 3 and 4, characterized by steatosis, inflammation and fibrosis, balloon cells, or Mallory bodies. Another recent paper has shown a high degree of correlation between types 3 and 4, such that these can be put together as one group representing 'NASH' [114]. The primary outcomes of cirrhosis, mortality, and liver-related mortality were determined with an average follow-up of 8 years.

The groups consisted of 49 type 1, 10 type 2, 19 type 3, and 54 type 4 subjects. Testing for hepatitis C virus (HCV) by polymerase chain reaction (PCR) in a subset of the biopsies excluded hepatitis C as a significant factor in most patients. No age or sex differences were noted between these groups. Combining types 1 and 2 and comparing these to the combined type 3 and 4 groups, the authors noted no difference in overall mortality, but a substantial difference in the frequency of cirrhosis was observed. Clinically defined cirrhosis developed much more commonly in the combined type 3–4 group (25%) than in the combined type 1–2 group (3%). In the combined type 3–4 group, the crude liver-related mortality rate was also higher than that in the combined type 1–2 group, and it was also substantially higher than the published crude death rate from United States census data.

The age of the patients with different types of NAFL warrants some additional comment. The similar age between the two major groups (type 1–2 versus type 3–4) suggests that these groups do not represent different stages in the evolution of NAFL, but rather, that they represent two distinct groups. In other words, it is unlikely that there is progression from type 1–2 over time to type 3–4. If there was such a progression, it can be reasoned that there would be either an age difference between the two groups (the more severely afflicted would be older) or there would be no detectable difference in the prognosis between the two groups. Thus, it is more likely that the individual who develops fatty infiltration of the liver, soon thereafter either controls the problem (through as yet inadequately understood mechanisms) and remains stable indefinitely, or the individual develops cellular injury manifested histologically as steatohepatitis.

Other studies support the validity of this classification scheme and its associated prognosis. Hilden et al. [115] reported on 58 patients with mild fatty liver followed for up 33 years. The study antedated the proposed classification scheme, but appears to have largely consisted of type 1 and 2 patients, since the presence of Mallory bodies was used as an exclusion criterion. Only one of these patients was known to have progressed to cirrhosis. In another retrospective study, Teli et al. [116] demonstrated similar results. They studied 40 patients with nonalcoholic steatosis and absent inflammation or fibrosis on the index biopsy (similar to type 1 NAFL). Although the inclusion of 6 patients with cancer-related cachexia and secondary steatosis limits the interpretation, the overall results were very similar to those noted above. None of the patients developed clinical cirrhosis. About one-half had persistent liver enzyme abnormalities, but among those undergoing repeat biopsy, only 1 showed the development of mild perivenular fibrosis after almost 10 years.

Lee [117] reported follow-up biopsy on 13 patients over an average of 3.5 years (1.2–6.9 years) after the baseline biopsy. Among these, 12 patients with features of NASH did not have cirrhosis at baseline. Follow-up histology revealed increased fibrosis in 5 and the development of cirrhosis in 2 patients. Similarly, Powell et al. [118] reported follow-up biopsy in 13 NASH patients with a median follow-up of 4.5 years. Repeat biopsy revealed worsening fibrosis in 3, progression to cirrhosis in 3, absent change in 6, and decreased fibrosis in 1. Of note, this study also demonstrated the progression of NASH with fibrosis or cirrhosis to cryptogenic cirrhosis with loss of the histological hallmarks of steatohepatitis. Bacon et al. [119] reported serial biopsy in 2 patients studied over approximately 5 years. One of these developed cirrhosis. Finally, Ratziu [120] reported serial biopsy in 14 patients with NAFL. Four of these had NASH at baseline, while 10 had only steatosis with minimal or no necroinflammatory activity or fibrosis. Among the 4 with baseline NASH (necroinflammatory activity and some degree of fibrosis), 1 progressed to cirrhosis over approximately 5 years, whereas none of the 10 patients without fibrosis progressed to cirrhosis.

Recent work has questioned some of the findings of older studies and raised new concerns. Harrison et al. [121] reported on 22 patients with NAFL followed with repeat biopsy over a mean of 5.7 years. Two patients with baseline biopsies showing simple steatosis were noted to develop mild degrees of fibrosis in follow-up biopsies performed 3–15 years after the baseline. Another interesting point from this work was that some patients had a relatively rapid change of fibrosis score between biopsies only several years apart. This suggests the possibility that NASH can remain stable for a long period of time and then show relatively rapid progression. Similar to prior studies, these authors noted a doubling in the percentage of patients with baseline fibrosis scores of stage 3 or 4 (bridging or cirrhosis) from 9% at baseline to 19% on follow-up.

Overall, it can be estimated that a substantial portion of NASH patients will remain stable or even improve, but about 40% will have worsening histology over approximately 5–7 years. As many as 20% develop worsening fibrosis, and up to 15%–20% progress to cirrhosis. Infrequently, the time over which the disease progresses will be considerably shorter than what we typically think. Possible explanations include rapid weight loss or possibly dietary composition, changes of which could precipitate deleterious changes in the fat-laden hepatocyte.

Mortality in NAFL

Among people with major risks for NAFL such as obesity and type 2 diabetes, liver-related mortality has largely been overshadowed by the high rate of cardio- and cerebrovascular death [122]. Nonetheless, obesity is a risk factor for cirrhosis-related death and hospitalization [123] and cirrhosis has been shown to be a common cause of death among type 2 diabetics [124]. In the latter study, the authors reported on mortality in 1939 type 2 diabetic patients followed for over 9 years. Not unexpectedly, vascular disease was the most common cause of death, with heart disease accounting for 19% of deaths, cerebrovascular disease for 16%, and renal disease for 13%. Cirrhosis was determined to be the cause of death in 6% of these patients, but the observed/expected ratio was actually higher (O/E = 2.67) for cirrhosis than for cerebro-cardiovascular disease overall (O/E = 2.12). This indicates a substantial risk for liver-related mortality in these patients, and suggests that liver-related morbidity is also likely to be an under-recognized factor in the management of diabetes and obesity.

Silent Morbidity of Advanced NASH in the Metabolic Syndrome

Cirrhosis is commonly recognized during the evaluation of some other problem in patients with longstanding obesity, type 2 diabetes, or hyperlipidemia [125]. The surprise discovery may occur during gallbladder surgery, during the evaluation of thrombocytopenia, or during the evaluation of new-onset gastrointestinal (GI) bleeding or ascites. Because cirrhosis fundamentally changes the physiology of the individual to that of the low systemic resistance (hyperdynamic) state, medication response is potentially altered; thus, common interventions may have unexpected side-effects. For instance, angiotensin-converting enzyme (ACE) inhibitors can promote salt retention and ascites formation. In addition, aspirin and other anti-thrombotic medications can promote fluid retention and/or GI bleeding (often from gastric antral vascular ectasia or 'GAVE'). The silent development of cirrhosis may also provide an alternative and potentially treatable explanation for certain symptoms. For instance, fatigue in the obese, diabetic patient with occult cirrhosis may actually reflect subclinical encephalopathy, treatable with typical ammonia-lowering regimens. Gut dysmotility, either as a result of associated diabetes or as part of NAFL [126], may contribute to constipation, making these patients especially prone to bouts of encephalopathy. Dyspnea may reflect the development of hepatopulmonary syndrome rather than intrinsic lung disease.

Given the potential role of the mitochondria in NASH (see below) [127, 128], it is interesting to further speculate upon the potential role of systemic mitochondrial dysfunction in the manifestations of NAFL. The existence of variation in mitochondrial integrity in different tissues offers a possible explanation. Mitochondrial heteroplasmy [129] could explain the susceptibility of different organs (such as the liver) to oxidative stress. A little-described ocular gaze disorder (intermittent disconjugate gaze or 'IDG'—seen in about 15% of NASH patients) lends support to the hypothesis [130]. Vision impairment is typically absent in IDG, but simple examination demonstrates disconjugate left or right lateral gaze that fluctuates in severity and may at times be undetectable, suggesting easy muscle fatigue as the likely mechanism.

Disease Modifiers and Confounding Variables

There are a number of variables which may alter the natural course of NAFL and which likely play some role in patients encountered day to day with this condition. Anti-diabetic agents, anti-lipidemic agents, dietary plans, exercise, over-the-counter herbal remedies, and modest ethanol use (which may actually be protective) are variables which have not been very well studied. Some of these have a potential role as therapy, but this is incompletely known (see below). Other agents, such as tamoxifen for breast cancer, amiodarone for cardiac dysrythmias, or methotrexate for psoriasis may accelerate cellular injury, and require careful consideration of the risk-benefit ratio. Coexisting NASH with other liver disease further introduces uncertainty into the evaluation of the fatty liver. Hepatitis C, especially genotype 3, is associated with some fatty infiltration, but frank NASH usually indicates the existence of risk factors for NAFL such as obesity and probably accelerates fibrosis [131]. We have also noted the development of NAFL in patients receiving steroids for autoimmune hepatitis. Its presence can be misleading, as it requires biopsy to differentiate from residual autoimmune inflammation.

Cryptogenic Cirrhosis

Cryptogenic cirrhosis—defined as cirrhosis of unknown cause after exhaustive diagnostic evaluation—remains a common problem, accounting for 5%–15% of cirrhosis patients in different series. While there are clearly a number of disease processes involved with the development of cryptogenic cirrhosis (including NASH, occult ethanol, subclinical autoimmune hepatitis, and non-B, non-C hepatitis), several studies have demonstrated a close association between NASH and cryptogenic cirrhosis. Based on the studies discussed below and a recent detailed histological analysis of explanted livers by Ayata et al. [132], it is estimated that NASH constitutes the underlying disease process in 30%–70% of cryptogenic cirrhosis patients.

The seminal observation linking cryptogenic cirrhosis and NASH was that of Elizabeth Powell and colleagues [133] in a 1990 report, in which serial biopsy of NASH patients demonstrated the loss of steatosis over years as the disease progressed from steatohepatitis with bridging fibrosis or cirrhosis to a stage of bland cirrhosis. The loss of steatosis in the regenerating nodules may result from altered blood flow from portosystemic shunting [134], capillarization of the sinusoids with loss of fenestrations, and secondary impairment of lipoprotein delivery, or a more fundamental alteration in hepatocyte fat metabolism.

Contos et al. [135] have published a useful descriptive scheme which divides patients with cryptogenic cirrhosis into two categories: those with inconclusive but suggestive features of NASH and those with 'bland' cirrhosis. Among 30 liver explants from [patients with] cryptogenic cirrhosis, 6 had absence of steatosis, but 24 had variable and patchy fatty infitration (mostly in the mild or 1+ range.) Twenty had Mallory hyaline and 21 had balloon cells. Seventeen of 30 had balloon degeneration, Mallory hyaline, and steatosis; 10 more had at least two of these features. Inflammatory changes were mild and mostly limited to the septae. Twenty-six of 30 had glycogenated nuclei (a finding considered corroborative of underlying and antecedent NASH.) The high prevalence of risk factors for NASH in these patients and the high recurrence rate following transplantation (nearly 100% by 5 years) supports the assertion that the majority of these cases represented progression of NASH.

We reported on a series of 70 consecutive patients with cryptogenic cirrhosis including both transplant and nontransplant candidates. Among these patients, 70% were female and 73% had a history of obesity and/or diabetes. These patients had an average age of 60 years, compared to 50 years for a control group of consecutive NASH patients, suggesting a 10-year interval of disease progression between NASH and cirrhosis. The prevalence of obesity and/or diabetes among the cirrhosis patients was not different from that in the NASH patients, but was significantly greater than that of age-matched patients with cirrhosis from hepatitis C or primary biliary cirrhosis (PBC). In many patients with cryptogenic cirrhosis, a past history of obesity may be hidden, due to weight loss associated with either aging or cirrhosis. A striking finding among the patients with cryptogenic cirrhosis was the fact that over half lacked major symptoms of portal hypertension; i.e., the cirrhosis was both cryptogenic and clinically silent. We also noted the common presence among both NASH and cryptogenic cirrhosis patients of a family history of unexplained liver disease—an association further supported by two additional publications [136, 137]. It was further noted that serum IgA was commonly elevated out of proportion to IgG. Serum IgA elevation, possibly as a result of lipid peroxidation and neoantigen formation, has long been associated with alcohol-induced steatohepatitis. A histologic study has also demonstrated deposition of IgA in liver tissue of both nonalcoholic and alcohol-related steatohepatitis [138]. Further studies are underway to examine serum and liver IgA as a marker of prior NASH in patients with cryptogenic cirrhosis.

Poonwalla et al. [139] published a report of 65 consecutive patients with cryptogenic cirrhosis awaiting liver transplantation. Each patient was compared to two age-matched control subjects with advanced cirrhosis from other etiologies and awaiting transplantation. The prevalence of obesity (55% versus 24%) and diabetes (47% versus 22%) was twice as high in the cryptogenic group as in the control group. Interestingly, the authors found no difference in the prevalence of hypercholesterolemia between the groups. Ong et al. [140] also reported on a series of 51 cryptogenic cirrhosis patients undergoing orthotopic liver transplantation (OLT). Similar to other series, the patients were commonly overweight females, and one-third had diabetes. Among the 25 patients undergoing post-transplant biopsy, 13 developed NAFL. Of these, 5 developed type 1 NAFL (simple steatosis) and 8 developed type 3–4 NAFL (NASH). Predictors of more severe histology post-OLT included diabetes, hypertriglyceridemia, and greater BMI. Possible interactions include the promotion of hepatic steatosis by glucocorticoids and the effects of cyclosporin A on the mitochondrial permeability transition pore.

Another perspective on this issue was provided by a report from Nair et al. [141], which demonstrated cryptogenic cirrhosis as the second most common cause of cirrhosis (after hepatitis C) among obese patients awaiting transplantation. However, because NASH patients who progress to cirrhosis often are much older (the median age in our series was 63 years) and frequently have comorbid conditions due to obesity, diabetes, and hyperlipidemia, their candidacy for transplantation is likely to be compromised. Thus, assessment of the significance of cryptogenic cirrhosis based on transplant lists is probably an underestimation, since many such patients are not considered for this intervention.

Cryptogenic Cirrhosis: Prognosis

The prognosis of obesity-related cryptogenic cirrhosis remains somewhat uncertain. However, grounds for increased concern regarding the development of complications of portal hypertension and hepatocellular cancer are slowly emerging. Ratziu et al. [142] recently compared the course of 27 overweight patients with cryptogenic cirrhosis to that of 10 lean patients with cryptogenic cirrhosis and 391 patients with hepatitis C-related cirrhosis in a retrospective follow-up cohort study. The prevalences of diabetes and hyperlipidemia were significantly higher in the obese cryptogenic compared to the lean cryptogenic cirrhosis group and the hepatitis C group. This difference persisted even when controlling for body mass index in the hepatitis C group. The mean age of the obese cryptogenic cirrhosis group was 62 years compared to 45 years for the lean cryptogenic group.

Most striking in this report was the fact that 9 of 27 obese cryptogenic patients were initially diagnosed with cirrhosis at the time of a major complication of portal hypertension, and 3 more had hepatocellular cancer at or near the time of the initial diagnosis of cirrhosis. After a mean follow-up of 22 months, 2 of the 15 patients presenting only with abnormal liver tests developed major complications of portal hypertension and 5 developed hepatocellular cancer. The authors concluded that obesity-related cirrhosis often diverges from the slow, indolent process characteristic of NASH and it may behave as aggressively as hepatitis C-related cirrhosis. The explanation for this observation remains uncertain, since loss of an active steatohepatitis would, intuitively, suggest a slowing of the process. Older age or perhaps accelerated parenchymal extinction [143] (a microvascular process) may offer an explanation.

Hepatocellular Cancer and NAFLD

The incidence of hepatocellular cancer has been increasing in the United States [144]. Although much of this has been attributed to hepatitis C, several papers have recently been published linking NAFL, insulin resistance, cryptogenic cirrhosis, and hepatocellular cancer [145]. Obesity itself has been implicated as a risk for various neoplasms [146]. Insulin resistance, associated hepatocyte hyperplasia, and decreased apoptosis have been implicated as factors in the development of hepatocellular cancer in ob/ob mice [147]. Diabetes has also been implicated as a factor in patients with viral hepatitis or alcoholic liver disease [148]. The observations in two recent case reports indicating hepatocellular cancer as a possible natural progression of NASH-related cirrhosis have subsequently been supported by larger studies (in addition to that of Ratziu et al. [142], noted above) [149, 150]. These two case reports (of one male, age 62, and one female, age 58—both with obesity and diabetes) described the development of hepatocellular cancer 6–10 years after the diagnosis of NASH was established by serological evaluation and biopsy.

Bugianesi et al. [151] reported on 23 patients with cryptogenic cirrhosis and hepatocellular cancer and compared this cohort to 115 age-matched controls from a registry of 641 cirrhosis-related hepatocellular cancers. A history of obesity (BMI > 30) was significantly more common in the cryptogenic group (41% versus 16%), as was a history of diabetes (50% versus 20%). The authors did not detect a difference in the duration of disease, the prevalence of genetic markers for hemochromatosis, or the character of the tumor (whether multifocal or metastatic). Compared to the overall group of hepatocellular cancer patients ($n = 641$), the cryptogenic cirrhosis group was older. However, in contrast to past series of cryptogenic cirrhosis patients, but similar to the paper of Ratziu et al. [142], there was a preponderance of males, suggesting an increased risk of hepatocellular cancer in males with cryptogenic cirrhosis.

In another report, Marrero et al. [152] reported the results of a prospective study on cirrhosis-related hepatocellular cancer. Among 105 patients with cirrhosis and hepatocellular cancer, 51% had hepatitis C as the underlying disease, but cryptogenic cirrhosis was the second most common association, accounting for 29% of the cases. The majority (58%) of these had a history of obesity, and 6 (20%) had documented prior steatohepatitis by biopsy performed an average of 4.5 years before the diagnosis of hepatocellular cancer. In contrast to the patients noted in prior series, these patients were mostly females, the tumors were often more advanced, and the patient was less likely to have undergone prior screening.

Pathogenesis of NAFL and NASH

Human fatty liver is a multifactorial disorder. Most likely, there are several different pathways by which one can arrive at a NASH, including the common metabolic syndrome patient with insulin resistance, toxin-induced fatty liver, such as Cotrim [2] has described in petrochemical workers, and possibly primary disorders of lipoprotein metabolism; for example, the fatty liver seen in kwashiorkor. Once fatty liver develops, there is some trigger that produces inflammation. Most likely this is lipid peroxidation, which serves as the 'second hit' proposed by James and Day [153]. However, further damage probably depends on additional variables, including genetic predisposition, nutritional status, exposure to toxins, exercise, and perhaps other less well-understood variables such as cold-exposure. Central to many of these variables is the functional status of the mitochondrion.

The Mitochondrion in NAFLD

Classically, mitochondrial disorders have included primarily neuromuscular diseases, many of which have been extensively characterized both clinically and physiologically [154]. Although cryptogenic cirrhosis has been described in patients with mitochondrial disease [155], liver disease in general or fatty liver in particular is rarely mentioned in the context of typical mitochondrial diseases. Nonetheless, a substantial body of literature has developed implicating mitochondrial dysfunction in various forms of hepatic steatosis [156]. The peculiar evolution of the mitochondrion from a free-living organism to an integral component of cell function may explain its relationship to cell death through apoptotic pathways [157]. Its role in fat metabolism and oxidative phosphorylation explains its role as both a source of free radicals and as a target for injury in oxidative stress [158].

The normal mitochondrion is a double-membrane organelle, numbering typically in the thousands per cell, with invaginations of the inner membrane which form cristae [159, 160]. The mitochondrial matrix contains enzymes responsible for the metabolism of amino acids (much of the AST elevation in steatohepatitis is mitochondrial in origin and presumably reflects injury to the organelle), as well as components of the tricarboxylic acid cycle, urea cycle, and heme synthesis pathway. In addition, the matrix contains 1–5 copies (up to 100 copies if replicating) of the mitochondrial genome organized into mitochondrial nuclei known as nucleoids [161]. Certain shapes are characteristic of different tissues—in liver, the tubular form is most common, while complex branching mitochondria are seen in skeletal muscle [162]. Variation in cristae (tubular in hepatocyte mitochondria, stacked in brown fat cells) and matrix density is seen between cell types.

The mitochondrial respiratory chain uses energy from the transport of electrons to generate an electrochemical gradient of protons (proton motive force, or PMF) across the inner mitochondrial membrane. Translocation of protons along the electrochemical gradient from the intermembrane space to the matrix through complex

V (ATP synthase) drives production of ATP. Uncoupling of oxidative phosphorylation, as in brown-fat mitochondria, results in the production of heat rather than ATP—an important function in thermogenesis. Opening of the mitochondrial transition pore also dissipates the electrochemical gradient, resulting in decreased ATP production. One percent to 2% of oxygen consumed during oxidative phosphorylation is only partially reduced, resulting in the formation of reactive oxygen species (ROS). These are primarily formed around ubiquinone of the respiratory chain (RC) and include superoxide anion and hydrogen peroxide (which can be converted to reactive hydroxyl ion). Mitochondrial superoxide dismutase and the selenium-dependant glutathione peroxidase serve to contain the ROS [163].

The Mitochondria in NAFL: Adaptation and Injury

Impaired oxidative phosphorylation and morphological changes of mitochondria in experimental steatosis were described roughly 50 years ago by Dianzani [164, 165]. Structural mitochondrial abnormalities characterized by enlargement and development of crystalline inclusions have been described in several forms of human fatty liver, including Wilson's disease [166], alcoholic steatohepatitis (where they were felt to be markers for early or less severe alcohol-related injury [167]), and nonalcoholic steatohepatitis (NASH) [168, 169]. Sanyal et al. [169] correlated the presence of these crystalline mitochondrial inclusions indirectly to oxidative stress. Once described as 'para'-crystalline, optical diffraction studies have demonstrated that the inclusions are in fact true crystals, although their composition remains uncertain [170]. From studies of NAFL patients in which we counted the number of megamitochondria in graded sections of electron microscope fields, we estimated that crystal-containing megamitochondria were seen in approximately 5%–15% of hepatocytes in NASH patients and in 5%–10% of the mitochondria within an afflicted cell [171]. The crystals occur as long parallel strands, each approximately 10 nm in diameter, with 20-nm spaces between strands. The 'sometimes seen' continuity with more normal-appearing cristae and the similarity of these structures to reversible lipid bilayers occurring in plants (etioplasts—precursors of chloroplasts) [172] and stress-induced structures in Amoeba mitochondria [173] suggests that these structures represent morphological or conformational changes in the cristae [174]. Similar structures containing bacterial DNA and a ferritin-like substance have also been observed in *Escherichia coli* exposed to a stress-induced protein (Dps) [175]. In spite of their pathological appearance, we were unable to demonstrate a relationship between the distribution of these structures and light microscopic changes, suggesting that they represent an adaptive response to oxidative injury [176].

These structural abnormalities are mirrored by disturbed ATP homeostasis, a likely result of impaired function of the mitochondrial electron transport chain. Dianzani [177] described decreased ATP and increased ADP in isolated mitochondria from rats with experimental fatty liver due to choline deficiency, CCL4 exposure, or white phosphorous exposure, and later demonstrated evidence of impaired oxidative-phosphorylation in experimental fatty liver. Rats fed choline-deficient diets developed fatty liver with increased mitochondrial lipid peroxides (Thiobarbituric reactive substances [TBARS] assay), decreased mitochondrial ATP, decreased ATP synthase activity, and markedly increased susceptibility to hepatic injury from starvation due to decreased glutathione levels [178]. The ability of betaine, an antioxidant, to reduce mitochondrial changes in CCL4-induced steatosis and the ability of gene delivery of superoxide dismutase in experimental fatty liver transplantation to likewise reduce injury further point to an association between mitochondrial morphological abnormalities, impaired ATP synthesis, and lipid peroxidation [179, 180].

The susceptibility of fatty livers to injury from ischemia-reperfusion also points to impaired ATP homeostasis [181]. Dysfunction for all components of the respiratory chain in hepatic mitochondria was demonstrated in a study of 38 NASH patients by Perez-Carrera et al. [182]. Respiratory chain activity was reduced to roughly 60% compared to identically processed controls in liver tissue homogenates normalized for volume to citrate synthase activity. Using an in vivo approach, Cortez-Pinto et al. [183] showed delayed recovery of hepatic ATP in patients with NAFL compared to controls following an intravenous fructose challenge using MR spectroscopy. Fructose, unlike glucose, requires an initial energy investment in the form of ATP prior to its subsequent metabolism. The authors of this study postulated that the intravenous bolus of fructose uncovered an energy deficit in the liver of patients with hepatic steatosis.

The physiological abnormalities in fatty liver include the expression of uncoupling protein 2 (UCP-2), which has been demonstrated experimentally in obese mice [184]. Uncoupling of the mitochondrial electron transport chain (ETC) is characteristic of thermogenic brown fat and shifts the energy of the ETC from ATP production to heat production. It has been suggested that this process represents a physiologic adaptation which reduces the formation of ROS [185], although the importance of this relationship has been questioned in terms of disease progression [186]. Mitochondrial uncoupling may be a direct result of increased free fatty acids in the intermitochondrial space [187], but because UCP-2 is normally produced only in fat tissue, its expression in the steatotic liver suggests that the fat-laden hepatocyte may not only look microscopically like an adipocyte but may also function essentially as such. We have recently noted that these similarities extend to the ultrastructural level [188] and suggested that the ballooned cell in NAFL is not always pathological but may be a form of adaptation to overabundant fat stores. In support of this, a recent abstract from Japan showed that markers for apoptosis, while seen in cells with microdroplet fat, did not appear to be invariable, suggesting that some cells successfully make a transition to a more stable unilocular fat-storing cell [189].

Fatty infiltration of solid organs, including the heart and liver, does exist in nature to meet the special metabolic demands imposed by migration, hibernation, or torpor. The best example occurs in some species of migratory ducks and geese. These birds undertake long migrations in a fasting state, and accumulate abundant fat in their liver prior to migration. This trait has been exploited commercially by human beings for the production of foie gras. Marked changes in apolipoprotein metabolism (decreased secretion of very low density lipoprotein [VLDL]) are seen in species which develop more substantial steatosis [190]. Rodents such as deer mice (genus Peromyscus) or ground squirrels that undergo periods of hibernation or daily torpor also accumulate fat in both their livers and their hearts. The California Desert mouse, adapted to the stressful conditions of desert life, develops steatosis and steatohepatitis in conditions of overabundant food availability [191]. It is speculated that these changes, adapted to feast and famine, provide both a ready source of metabolic fuel and a means of heat production—an essential function in cold-adapted homeothermic organisms, but potentially pathological in the overfed state [192].

Recently, a link between dietary thermogenesis, obesity, sympathetic nervous system activity, and cold exposure has been described [193, 194]. It is thought that the balance between dietary intake and cold exposure (or some other stress) influences both basal metabolic and facultative (in response to cold exposure) thermogenesis by acting through the sympathetic nervous system, which influences the expression of UCP in brown fat. The role of adrenergic stimulation in steatohepatitis in ObOb mice seems relevant to this process [195]. A similar process may be present in some rudimentary fashion in higher mammals, and could explain some of the familial [196, 197] and ethnic [198] variation described in human NAFL.

Variation in mitochondrial DNA susceptibility to oxidative stress could also play a role in variable tissue injury. Injury probably depends on a threshold effect depending on the energy needs of tissue [199–201]. The lack of substantial repair machinery in the mitochondria is thought to contribute to their increased susceptibility to oxidative injury and the accumulation of mtDNA mutations and/or deletions that eventually lead to impaired cellular respiration and cell death. In NASH patients, a 5-kb gene deletion (the 'common' deletion associated with Kearns-Sayer mitochondrialopathy) was detected in liver tissue of 1 in 5 patients tested in one series and in 10 of 14 patients in another series [203]. Another patient in the latter series expressed the 8344 mutation seen in the myoclonic epilepsy and ragged red fibers (MERRF) syndrome.

Hepatic steatosis and cryptogenic cirrhosis may be seen in specific mitochondrial gene mutations and deletions [204, 205]. Symmetrical lipomatosis, or Madelungs disease [206], which is characterized by obesity, lipomatosis, insulin resistance, and dyslipidemia has been associated with mitochondrial DNA mutation 8344, which also is evident in MERFF syndrome [207]. Another mitochondrial mutation (3243, seen also in MELAS syndrome—mitochondrial encephalopathy, lactic acidosis, and stroke-like episodes) has been associated with MIDD (maternally inherited diabetes and deafness) [208]. Neither the prevalence of fatty liver in these patients nor the prevalence of these mutations in NASH are known. However, it has been estimated that 1%–2% of type 2 diabetes patients harbor the nt-3243 mutation [209].

Apoptotic bodies are occasionally seen in NASH at light microscopy and probably represent the result of mitochondrial injury and imbalance of pro- versus anti-apoptotic factors. Their infrequent presence by light microscopy, in comparison to their presence in alcohol-related liver injury [210], is consistent with the typically slower rate of clinical progression of NASH compared to alcoholic steatohepatitis (ASH). Mitochondrial swelling, outer membrane rupture, and extrusion of inner matrix material have been observed in mouse hepatocytes after stimulation of apoptosis by FAS activation [211]. Recently, it was shown that more subtle signs of apoptosis (evident by the terminal deoxynucleotidyl transferase (TdT)-mediated dUTP-biotin nick end labeling [TUNEL] assay) were increased in patients with NASH relative to control patients [212]. This was accompanied by increased activated caspase and FAS—both factors in the cascade leading to apoptosis. Agents thought to potentiate or stimulate the opening of the mitochondrial permeability transition (MPT) pore include reactive oxygen species in oxidative stress, Bax, tumor necrosis factor (TNF), and ceramide. Both pro-apoptotic (Bax) and anti-apoptotic (Bcl-2, Bcl-xl) factors are increased in experimental models of fatty liver [213].

The association of partial lipodystrophy, a disorder of peripheral fat metabolism, and NAFL provides perhaps the most apparent clinical example of NAFL as a systemic disorder of fat metabolism [214]. Mitochondrial heteroplasmy (the uneven dispersion of weak and susceptible mitochondria in different tissues—see above) combined with environmental influences (such as dietary composition, exercise levels, and aging) and the metabolic demands of different tissues could explain the variable expression of a latent systemic disorder. Degonl et al. [215] have suggested that genetic variation in the trafficking of superoxide dismutase into the mitochondria may explain, to some extent, individual variation in susceptibility to oxidative injury in alcohol-related liver disease.

Skeletal muscle mitochondrial dysfunction was implicated, using MR spectroscopy, in the development of age-related insulin resistance [216]. The authors further speculated that mitochondrial injury could play a role in the development of islet cell failure associated with progression from silent hyperinsulinemia to frank type 2 diabetes in obese patients. Dietary fatty acid composition has also been implicated in skeletal muscle insulin sensitivity [217]. The lipotoxicity hypothesis may explain some aspects of cellular toxicity in conditions of excess body fat. Central to this hypothesis is the potential role of ceramide, an acylated sphingosine (derived from palmitic acid) and intermediate substance in the synthesis of sphingomyelin, which can activate mitochondrial-stimulated apoptosis. Recent gene chip microarray assays examining the hepatic expression of mRNA in NASH [218] indicated that potentially toxic fatty acids and weak or senescent mitochondria, coupled with deficient mitochondrial antioxidant systems (superoxide dismutase and catalase) could explain the development of cellular failure in many different organs, especially those with high basal metabolic rates.

Current Therapy of NAFL: General Considerations

Other than perhaps exercise and diet, there is no universally agreed upon treatment, and therapeutic strategies have been largely empirical because the pathogenesis remains uncertain in many respects. A number of papers have been published reviewing current therapy. Below, we provide a summary of some of the salient points regarding therapy [219–223]. Because NAFL is usually associated with the comorbid conditions of type II diabetes, obesity, and/or hypertryglyceridemia, treatment of these conditions is often a consideration. Other important general considerations include the issue of alcohol prohibition versus moderation to levels less than 20 g/day. Data indicating a protective effect of modest ethanol ingestion in both diabetes and NAFL support a moderate position on this [224, 225]. A pragmatic recommendation is to tailor the recommendation to the histology, with abstinence if significant fibrosis has already developed. The use of medications that may promote steatohepatitis (e.g., glucocorticoids, amiodarone, methotrexate, or tamoxifen) also requires consideration and the weighing of the risks and benefits of liver injury. Unfortunately, there are often no clear guidelines when making these recommendations. We frequently suggest the use of vitamin E, ursodiol, or ubiquinone in this setting, although data are also lacking. Another increasingly common but little-explored issue is workplace exposure to solvents [226–228]. A part of treatment may necessitate measures to reduce or eliminate exposure, especially if fibrosis is evident on biopsy. Finally, if cirrhosis is proven or suspected in a NAFL patient, a review of medications with potential adverse effects in the cirrhotic patient (e.g., aspirin, other non-steroidal anti-inflammatory drugs, and angiotensin-converting enzyme inhibitors) is warranted.

Exercise, Diet, and Weight Loss

Exercise Alone

Exercise and diet form a cornerstone of therapy [229]. Although it is difficult to clearly separate exercise from weight loss, the concept of the 'fit fat' individual (i.e., relatively well conditioned but obese) suggests a benefit to exercise in the absence of weight loss [230]. Further studies examining the lactate threshold and exercise oxygen consumption are needed to assess the role of 'conditioning' exercise.

Exercise, Diet, and Weight Loss

There are a number of small reports of combined diet and exercise therapies in both adults and children. These typically reveal improved biochemical parameters, but variable changes in histology [231–243]. Some of these diets included unrealistic and severe calorie restriction. It is also important to note that histological exacerbation has been observed with rapid weight loss [244]. This is thought to result from an increase in the flow of free fatty acids to the liver from the mesenteric fat stores, resulting in increased lipid peroxidation. Protein malnutrition with impaired export of apoprotein fat from the liver and micronutrient deficiency could also play a role. Recently, a more practical 15-month lifestyle modification plan, including dietary changes and exercise in 31 patients showed success in loss of weight in 68% [245]. Among these patients, the authors noted a significant relationship between decreased ALT and the degree of weight loss and reduction in fibrosis in 7 of 14 undergoing repeat biopsy.

Exercise alters substrate utilization in skeletal muscle and insulin sensitivity, although obese individuals may be resistant to these changes [246, 247], and only about one-third of patients achieve target levels of exercise [248–250]. Higher intensity exercise regimens are probably more effective in producing significant metabolic changes [251]. Intermittent exercise also has been found to be as effective as daily exercise in a randomized controlled study involving obese women [252]. Both aerobic and resistance exercise have been shown to have some benefit in reducing weight [253]. Another novel metabolic approach is the use of hyperthermia, which has been noted to alter hepatic steatosis in patients undergoing experimental treatment for hepatitis C [254]. A contrasting approach is that of cold exposure, popularly known as 'kniepering'. A physiologic basis for this approach may lie in experimental work showing altered thermogenesis in cold-exposed animals [255, 256].

Popular Diets

The effects on the fatty liver of many popular diets, such as the Zone or Atkins diet [257, 258], are not known, although a recent abstract suggested that reduced carbohydrate intake may be of benefit [259]. The metabolic changes induced by the low carbohydrate-high protein diet warrant some additional concern and perhaps precaution, as the fatty liver is prone to increased production of ketone bodies. A pragmatic approach is to recommend a reduced calorie, balanced diet such as that endorsed by the National Heart, Lung, and Blood Institute (NHLBI) and National Institute of Diabetes, Digestive and Kidney Disease [NIDDK] [260], the American Heart Association [261], the American Diabetes Association [262], or the low glycemic index diet which emphasizes dietary composition [263].

Dietary Supplements

The effects on the liver of dietary supplements have been well investigated. Increased polyunsaturated fatty acids (PUFA; fish, and flax seed oils) alter insulin sensitivity and prostaglandin metabolism, may increase UCP (uncoupling protein) expression, and may promote lipid peroxidation, but the net effect in steatohepatitis is not known [264–272]. Dietary fructans, but not cellulose, decreased triglyceride accumulation in the liver of obese Zucker rats [273], and, likewise, warrant further study. Appetite-suppressing agents have lost favor due to their side-effects [274, 275]. However, a potential role for orlistat (tetrahydrolipostatin), a lipase inhibitor, was noted in a study of ten patients with proven NASH who underwent 6 months of orlistat therapy. Normalization of transaminases in six patients, weight reduction, and mild but potentially significant improvement in steatosis and fibrosis were seen [276]. Malabsorption of vitamin E is a relevant concern with fat-malabsorbing agents. Phentermine and sibutramine, possibly effective in achieving weight loss, are of uncertain benefit in NAFL [277]. In light of the concept of the liver as a normal fat-storing organ (see above), agents that produce lipoatrophy may be of particular safety concern.

Surgical Weight Loss

Increasingly, patients who fail diet and exercise-based regimens are turning to surgical therapy. Several studies have reported beneficial effects of bariatric surgery [278–282]. Proximal gastric bypass has now largely replaced vertical-banded gastroplasty as well as the older jejunoileal bypass. Several of these studies have reported benefits in both hepatic histology and general parameters of the metabolic syndrome, and a recent report of post-transplantation NASH noted normalization of liver enzymes, lipids, and glucose, with histological regression of steatosis after weight loss from a Roux-en-Y gastric bypass [283]. Precipitous weight loss, however, has the potential to severely exacerbate steatohepatitis. Preoperative treatment with cytoprotective or anti-oxidant agents has not been tested but is sometimes recommended. Prior studies in the now discarded intestinal bypass procedure further support a role for antibiotics and amino-acid supplementation for patients who experience decompensation [284, 285].

Cytoprotective and Antioxidant Agents

Ursodeoxycholic acid (ursodiol or UDCA) has been studied extensively in other liver diseases and has shown promise in preliminary studies of its use in NAFLD [286–290]. Laurin et al. [291] compared UDCA to clofibrate in 40 patients over a year of therapy. They showed improvement of the liver enzymes as well as histological grade of steatosis in the UDCA group, but no change in fibrosis. The results of a randomized, multicenter trial (K.D. Lindor et al. [292]) are soon to be available. Preliminary results suggest that UDCA alone will not be sufficient to cause regression of NASH, although, based on its safety and the results of earlier studies, further investigation is warranted to assess its role as a co-factor with other agents such as vitamin E.

Early reports have shown that taurine, given to rats with ethanol-induced hepatic steatosis, normalized liver enzymes and improved steatosis [293–296]. The protective effects of taurine were attributed to the potential of bile acids, especially taurine-conjugated bile acids (taurocholic acid) to inhibit the activity of some microsomal enzymes (CYP2E1). A small study of ten children with fatty liver noted improved ALT and steatosis measured on CT [297]. Triacetyl uridine is a potentially important cytoprotective agent in experimental choline-deficient rats, but has not been tested in humans [298]. Lecithin increases plasma free choline and decreases hepatic steatosis in patients on long-term total parenteral nutrition, and other patients [299, 300].

Vitamin E has had positive effects in both experimental and human fatty liver [301–303]. Its excellent safety profile favors its use in NAFL, although caution is warranted in patients with prior coronary artery disease, in whom vitamin E is associated with blunted efficacy of statin drugs [304]. Less impressive results were seen in one study of combination antioxidants [305]. However, a recent controlled trial compared vitamin E, given for 1 year in 22 patients with various degrees of NAFL. Therapy was associated with reduction of ALT, modest improvement of steatosis and inflammation, and a significant reduction in the level of plasma transforming growth factor-β1, which has been implicated in the development of hepatic fibrosis [306]. Another recent randomized, placebo-controlled, double-blind study of vitamin E (1000 U) and vitamin C (1000 mg) demonstrated a significant reduction in fibrosis in the treated group [307].

Agents that potentiate the transmethylation pathways and augment the synthesis of glutathione (GSH) have undergone study. In animal studies with alcoholic-induced hepatic steatosis, S-adenosyl-methionine (SAM) replenished mitochondrial reduced GSH [308–310]. It was also shown that SAM significantly increased cytoslic and mitochondrial GSH in ischemic-reperfused steatotic rats [311–313]. Human studies with SAM in chronic liver disease have also been encouraging [314–316]. Betaine, a naturally occurring metabolite of choline, and a methyl donor in an alternative pathway for re-methylation of homocysteine to methionine, was studied in a small trial involving 10 NASH patients for 1 year [317, 318]. Transaminase normalized in 3, decreased in 3, and was unchanged in 1 of the 7 patients who completed the study. Improvement in the degree of steatosis and in necroinflammatory grade was noted. Miglio et al. [319] studied 191 patients with NAFL treated with an oral form of betaine glucuronate combined with diethanolamine glucuronate and nicotinamide ascorbate. They noted improvement in hepatic steatosis, hepatomegaly, and aminotransferases. *N*-Acetylcysteine (NAC) has been studied in animal models with hepatic steatosis [320, 321]. A small human study of 11 NASH patients, managed initially with diet regulation followed by NAC therapy, showed improvement in aminotransferases [322].

Other miscellaneous agents with purported or suspected antioxidant effects include silymarin [323]; this is a milk thistle derivative commonly used by patients, although we are not aware of published studies of its use in NAFL. Others in this category include histamine, which possesses indirect antioxidant properties [324], and the 21-aminosteroids, a group of substances known as lazaroids, which may warrant pilot work [325]. Probiotics have shown promise in an animal model, in which Li et al. [326] showed that treatment with VSL#3 (a probiotic preparation) reduced hepatic total fatty content, and decreased serum ALT levels. The authors conjectured that these results supported the concept that intestinal bacteria induce signals that play a role in hepatic insulin resistance and NAFLD [326]. Less is known about the potential effects of selenium, β-carotene, ubiquinone (Co-Q), ethanolamines, niacinamide, glucosamine, chondroitin, vitamin B complexes, vitamin C, and lipoic acid, all agents with purported antioxidant effects.

Anti-Diabetic and Insulin-Sensitizing Agents

All of these agents represent a step up in the level of therapy above the mild side-effect profiles of the cytoprotective or antioxidant agents and thus will likely be restricted to patients with type 3–4 NAFL. Insulin, sometimes recommended early in the course of type II diabetes [327], and sulfonylureas have not been adequately addressed for their effects on the liver in patients with NAFL.

The newer class of agents known as thiazolidinediones (TZD) have been studied to some extent, and early work shows their promise as therapeutic agents in NAFL [328–334]. These agents stimulate nuclear transcription factors [335], alter skeletal muscle glucose uptake (through increased GLUT4 activity) [336], decrease central adiposity [337], promote adipocyte differentiation, alter mitochondrial mass [338], and alter thermogenesis [339]. The efficacy of troglitazone in lipodystrophy suggests a primary effect on lipid metabolism and basal metabolism, since the respiratory quotient (RQ) is altered [340]. We previously demonstrated a reduction in inflammatory and fatty infiltration after a short course (3–6 months) of troglitazone, with no change in apoptosis markers. This agent has been withdrawn due to rare but potentially fatal idiosyncratic hepatotoxicity. However, pioglitazone and rosiglitazone, in two controlled studies, by Sanyal [341] and Tetri [342], have also shown reduction in inflammation and steatosis, as well as fibrosis. The effect on adipocyte differentiation probably explains the shift in adiposity from central solid-organ deposition (including liver) to peripheral fat stores in all human studies to date. Although hepatic effects subside after therapy is stopped, the effect on peripheral fat stores appears to be a lasting effect, as weight gain during therapy appears to persist after discontinuation of the medication [343]. This is of obvious concern and will limit the overall utility of these agents.

Metformin has undergone limited but promising studies in experimental and human NAFL [344–347]. It appears to divert fatty acids from triglyceride production to mitochondrial beta oxidation [348]. Data regarding histological response in human NAFL is very limited, but one report, by Ahmet Uygen et al. (personal communication) has shown histological improvement in a necroinflammatory index, although details of this report are not yet available. Other candidate agents include acarbose [an α-glucosidase inhibitor) [349], acipimox (inhibits lipolysis) [350], and d-chiro-inositol [351].

Anti-Hyperlipidemic Agents

Fibrates altered lipoprotein activity through the PPAR-α receptor, but had no histological effects in an early report by Laurin et al. [352]. However, bezafibrate has since shown benefit in tamoxifen-associated steatohepatitis in one very small pilot study [353]. In addition, Basaranoglu et al. [354] showed improvement in liver enzymes in a study of gemfibrozil, but histology was not measured. The hydroxymethylglutaryl-Co-enzyme A (HMG-CoA) reductase inhibitors, commonly known as statins, are becoming increasingly popular agents for the treatment of hypercholesterolemia, but their risk-benefit profile in fatty liver remains ill-defined [355]. A pilot study has shown improvement in biochemical and histological parameters in a small sample of patients treated with atorvastatin, and another recent report showed no significant histologic differences between controls and patients using various statin drugs [356, 357]. However, a report of these drugs, subclinical skeletal muscle toxicity, characterized by the formation of ragged red fibers and mediated by mitochondrial injury [358], is justifiable cause for concern for their longterm use in NAFL and raises concern for silent liver injury. The potential injurious effects of 'statin' drugs is emphasized by the potential role of apoprotein metabolism in NAFL [359, 360]. Other lipid-lowering agents such as colesevelam or other resin-binding agents have not been investigated. Dietary changes, such as supplementation with polyunsaturated fats, are discussed above.

Treatment of Secondary Causes of Hepatic Steatosis

Abnormal iron indices without frank hemochromatosis have been reported (see above). Iron deposition could be detrimental in NAFL due to the pro-oxidant effects of iron. One study has shown improvement in liver enzymes and insulin sensitivity in a group of *HFE* gene-negative patients treated with serial phlebotomy for iron reduction [361]. Whether this form of therapy has general applicability or is better reserved for patients with evidence of iron overload remains to be seen. Hepatitis C has been associated with steatosis, especially in patients with genotype 3a [362–367]. Recent studies have shown improvement of steatosis in chronic hepatitis C patients after successful antiviral therapy [368–370]. On the other hand, Hickman et al. [371] showed improvement of liver histology in chronic hepatitis C patients after weight reduction alone. This remains to be resolved. A secondary form of NASH may be seen in steroid-treated patients—it can be confused with persistent autoimmune hepatitis. This has resolved after the withdrawal of the medication. Other secondary forms of NAFL, such as that associated with tamoxifen, may be ameliorated by the addition of anti-oxidants or cytoprotective agents, as noted above, but this remains conjectural.

Liver Transplantation

NAFL patients who progress to cirrhosis are often poor candidates for transplantation, due to comorbid conditions. However, in the United States, firm guidelines do not exist to exclude these patients from transplantation, although it is known that the results of transplantation in obese patients are not as good as those in relatively lean patients [372]. Both the *recurrence* of NASH, in patients with previously established NASH leading to cirrhosis [373–376], and the *occurrence* of NASH, following transplantation for cryptogenic cirrhosis [377, 378], have been reported. Progression to steatohepatitis and subsequently to cirrhosis in the graft may be seen, although predictive factors and treatment have not been well defined. Immunosuppression could play a role, due to the promotion of fatty liver and diabetes with corticosteroid use, and could have more direct effects, such as the effect of cyclosporine on the mitochondrion [379].

References

1. Matteoni CA, Younossi ZM, Gramlich T, Boparai N, Liu YC, McCullough AJ (1999) Nonalcoholic fatty liver disease: a spectrum of clinical and pathological severity. Gastroenterology 116: 1413–1419
2. Cotrim HP, De Freitas LA, Freitas C, Braga L, Sousa R, Carvalho F, Parana R, Santos-Jesus R, Andrade NASH in workers exposed to chemicals with or without associated metabolic conditions. Liver Int 2004
3. Morgan W (1877) The Liver and its Diseases, Both Functional and Organic. Their History, Anatomy, Chemistry, Pathology, Physiology, and Treatment. Homoeopathic, London, University of Virginia Historical Collection, p 144
4. Tumen HJ, Cohn EM (1946) Cirrhosis. In: Bockus HL (ed) Gastroenterology, vol. III. Saunders, Philadelphia, pp 385–392
5. Zelman S (1958) The liver in obesity. Arch Intern Med 90: 141–156
6. Faloon WW (1988) Hepatobiliary effects of obesity and weight-reducing surgery. Semin Liver Dis 8: 229–236
7. Ludwig J, Viggiano TR, McGill DB, Ott BJ (1980) Nonalcoholic steatohepatitis. Mayo Clin Proc 55: 434–438
8. Sanyal AJ (2002) AGA technical review on nonalcoholic fatty liver disease. Gastroenterology 123: 1705–1725
9. Cairns SR, Peters TJ (1983) Biochemical analysis of hepatic lipid in alcoholic and diabetic and control subjects. Clin Sci 65: 645–652
10. James OFW (2002) NASH/NAFLD Management. AASLD Single Topic Conference on NASH Syllabus, Atlanta, Georgia
11. Bellentani S, Saccoccio G, Masutti F, Croce LS, Brandi G, Sasso F, Cristanini G, Tiribelli C (2000) Prevalence of and risk factors for hepatic steatosis in Northern Italy. Ann Intern Med 132: 112–117
12. Clark JM, Brancati FL, Diehl AM (2001) Nonalcoholic fatty liver disease: the most common cause of abnormal liver enzymes in the US population (abstract). Gastroenterology 120: 65
13. Nomura H, Kashiwagi S, Hayashai J, Kujiyama W, Tani S, Goto M (1988) Prevalence of fatty liver in a general population of Okinawa, Japan. Jpn J Med 27: 142–149
14. Siegelman ES, Rosen MA (2001) Imaging of steatosis. Semin Liver Dis 21: 71–80
15. Van der Kooy K, Seidell JC (1993) Techniques for the measurements of visceral fat: a practical guide. Int J Obes 17: 187–196

16. Saadeh S, Younossi ZM, Remer EM, Gramlish T, Ong JP, Hurley M, Mullen KD, Cooper JN, Sheridan MJ (2002) The utility of radiological imaging in nonalcoholic fatty liver disease. Gastroenterology 123: 745–750
17. Celle G, Savarino V, Picciotto A, Magnolia MR, Scalabrini P, Dodero M (1988) Is hepatic ultrasonography a valid alternative tool to liver biopsy? Report on 507 cases studied with both techniques. Dig Dis Sci 33: 467–471
18. Quinn SF, Gosink BB (1985) Characteristic sonographic signs of hepatic fatty infiltration. AJR Am J Roentgenol 145: 753–755
19. Jacobs JE, Birnbaum BA, Shapiro MA, Langlotz CP, Slosman F, Rubesin SE, Horii SC (1998) Diagnostic criteria for fatty infiltration of the liver on contrast enhanced helical CT. AJR Am J Roentgenol 171: 659–664
20. Levenson H, Greensite F, Hoefs J, Friloux L, Applegate G, Silva E, Kanel G, Buxton R (1991) Fatty infiltration of the liver: quantification with phase-contrast MR imaging at 1.5 T vs biopsy. AJR Am J Roentgenol 156: 307–312
21. Cortez-Pinto H, Chatham J, Chacko VP, Arnold C, Rashid A, Diehl AM (1999) Alterations in liver ATP homeostasis in human nonalcoholic steatohepatitis: a pilot study. JAMA 282: 1659–1664
22. Hilden M, Juhl E, Thomsen AC, Christoffersen P (1973) Fatty liver persisting for up to 33 years. Acta Med Scand 194: 485–489
23. Teli MR, James OFW, Burt AD, Bennett MK, Day CP (1995) The natural history of nonalcoholic fatty liver: a followup study. Hepatology 22: 1714–1719
24. Harrison SA, Torgerson S, Hayashi PH (2003) The natural history of nonalcoholic fatty liver disease: a clinical histopathological study. Am J Gastroenterol 98: 2042–2047
25. Powell EE, Cooksley WG, Hanson R, Searll J, Halliday JW, Powell LW (1990) The natural history of nonalcoholic steatohepatitis: a follow-up study of 42 patients for up to 21 years. Hepatology 11: 74–80
26. Caldwell SH, Oelsner DH, Iezzoni JC, Hespenheide EE, Battle EH, Driscoll CJ (1999) Cryptogenic cirrhosis: clinical characterization and risk factors for underlying disease. Hepatology 29: 664–669
27. Poonawala A, Nair SP, Thuluvath PJ (2000) Prevalence of obesity and diabetes in patients with cryptogenic cirrhosis: a case-control study. Hepatology 32: 689–692
28. Mendiola AE, Gish RG (2001) Risk factors for NASH in patients with cryptogenic cirrhosis (abstract). Gastroenterology 120: 545
29. Contos MJ, Cales W, Sterling RK, Lukeric VA, Shiffman ML, Mills AS, Fisher RA, Ham J, Sanyal AJ (2001) Development of nonalcoholic fatty liver disease after orthotopic liver transplantation for cryptogenic cirrhosis. Liver Transpl 7: 363–373
30. Ayata G, Gordon FD, Lewis WD, Pomfret E, Pomposelli JJ, Jenkins RL, Khettry U (2002) Cryptogenic cirrhosis: clinicopathologic findings at and after liver transplantation. Hum Pathol 33: 1098–1104
31. Basaranoglu M, Ozbay G, Caldwell SH, Sonsuz A (2003) Refinement of a clinicopathological typing system for NAFLD (abstract). Hepatology 34: 505A
32. Brunt EM, Janney CG, Di Bisceglie AM, Neuschwander-Tetri BA, Bacon BR (1999) Nonalcoholic steatohepatitis: a proposal for grading and staging the histologic lesions. Am J Gastroenterol 94: 2467–2474
33. Mendler MH, Yashar B, Govindarajan S, Kanel G (2002) A novel semi-quantitative histological scoring system for non-alcoholic fatty liver disease: evaluation and clinical correlations (abstract). Hepatology 36: 407
34. Navarro VJ, St Louis T, Bell BZ, Sofair AN (2003) Chronic liver disease in the primary care practices of Waterbury, Connecticut. Hepatology 38: 1062–1063
35. Marchesini G, Bugianesi E, Forlani G, Cerrelli F, Lenzi M, Manini R, Natale S, Vanni E, Villanova N, Melchionda N, Rizzetto M (2003) Nonalcoholic fatty liver steatohepatitis, and the metabolic syndrome. Hepatology 37: 917–923
36. Neuschwander-Tetri BA, Caldwell SH (2003) Nonalcoholic steatohepatitis: summary of an AASLD single topic conference. Hepatology 37: 1202–1219

37. Assy N, Kaita K, Mymin D, Levy C, Rosser B, Minuk G (2000) Fatty infiltration of liver in hyperlipidemic patients. Dig Dis Sciences 45: 1929–1934
38. Rashid M, Roberts EA (2000) Nonalcoholic steatohepatitis in children. J Pediatr Gastroenterol Nutr 30: 48–53
39. Struben VMD, Hespenheide EE, Caldwell SH (2000) Familial patterns of non-alcoholic steatohepatitis and cryptogenic cirrhosis. Am J Med 108: 9–13
40. Willner IR, Waters B, Patil SR, Reuben A, Morelli J, Riely CA (2001) Ninety patients with nonalcoholic steatohepatitis: insulin resistance, familial tendency and severity of disease. Am J Gastroenterol 96: 2957–2961
41. Cortez-Pinto H, Camilo ME, Baptista A, de Oliveira AG, De Moura MC (1999) Non-alcoholic fatty liver: another feature of the metabolic syndrome. Clin Nutr 18: 353–358
42. Knobler H, Schatter A, Zhornicki T, Malnick SD, Keter D, Sokolovsaya N, Lurie Y, Bass DD (19999) Fatty liver—an additional and treatable feature of the insulin resistance syndrome. QJM 92: 73–79
43. Ikai E, Ishizaki M, Suzuki Y, Ishida M, Noborizaka Y, Yamada Y (1995) Association between hepatic steatosis, insulin resistance, and hyperinsulinemia as related to hypertension in alcohol consumers and obese people. J Hum Hypertens 9: 101–105
44. Lobo RA, Carmino E (2000) The importance of diagnosing the polycystic ovary syndrome. Ann Intern Med 132: 989–993
45. Kuczmarski RJ, Carroll MD, Flegal KM, Troiano RP (1997) Varying body mass index cutoff points to describe overweight prevalence among US adults: NHANES III (1988 to 1994). Obesity Res 5: 542–548
46. NHLBI Obesity Task Force (1998) Clinical guidelines on the identification, evaluation, and treatment of overweight and obesity in adults—the evidence report. Obesity Res 6(Suppl 2): 51S–209S
47. Lee JH, Rhee PL, Lee JK, Lee KT, Kim JJ, Koh KC, Paik SW, Rhee JC, Choi KW (1998) Role of hyperinsulinemia and glucose intolerance in the pathogenesis of nonalcoholic fatty liver in patients with normal body weight. Korean J Intern Med 13: 12–14
48. Banerji MA, Faridi N, Atluri R, Chaiken RL, Lebovitz HE (1999) Body composition, visceral fat, leptin, and insulin resistance in Asian Indian men. J Clin Endocrinol Metab 84: 137–144
49. Pagano G, Pacini G, Musso G, Gambino R, Mecca F, Depetris N, Cassader M, David E, Cavallo-Perin P, Rizzetto M (2002) Nonalcoholic steatohepatitis, insulin resistance and metabolic syndrome: further evidence for an etiologic association. Hepatology 35: 367–372
50. Chitturi S, Abeygunasekera S, Farrell GC, Holmes-Walker J, Hui JM, Fung C, Karim R, Lin R, Samarasinghe D, Liddle C, Weltman M, George J (2002) NASH and insulin resistance: insulin hypersecretion and specific association with the insulin resistance syndrome. Hepatology 35: 373–379
51. Pouliot MC, Despres JP, Lemieux S, Moorjani S, Bouchard C, Tremblay A, Nadeau A, Lupien PJ (1994) Waist circumference and abdominal sagittal diameter: best simple anthropometric indices of abdominal visceral adipose tissue accumulation and related cardiovascular risk in men and women. Am J Cardiol 73: 460–468
52. Ong JP, Hazem E, Younoszai A, Goodman Z, Grant G, Christensen A, Chandhoke V, Cooper J, Bopari N, Younossi ZM (2002) Predictors of non-alcoholic steatohepatitis and fibrosis in non-alcoholic fatty liver disease (abstract). Hepatology 36: 407
53. Kuczmarski RJ (1989) Need for body composition information in elderly subjects. Am J Clin Nutr 50: 1150–1157
54. Andersen T, Gluud C (1984) Liver morphology in morbid obesity: a literature study. Int J Obes 8: 97–106
55. Andersen T, Christoffersen P, Gluud C (1984) The liver in consecutive patients with morbid obesity: a clinical, morphological and biochemical study. Int J Obes 8: 107–115

56. Ratziu V, Giral P, Charlotte F, Bruckert E, Thibault V, Theodorou I, Khalil L, Turpin G, Opolon P, Poynard T (2000) Liver fibrosis in overweight patients. Gastroenterology 118: 1117–1123
57. Garcia-Monzon C, Martin-Perez E, Iacono OL, Fernandez-Bermejo M, Majano PL, Apolinario A, Larranaga E, Moreno-Otero R (2000) Characterization of pathogenic and prognostic factors of nonalcoholic steatohepatitis associated with obesity. J Hepatol 33: 716–724
58. Braillon A, Capron JP, Herve MA, Degott C, Quenum C (1985) Liver in obesity. Gut 26: 133–139
59. Marchesini G, Brizi M, Morselli-Labate AM, Bianchi G, Bugianesi E, McCullough AJ, Forlani G, Melchionda N (1999) Association of nonalcoholic fatty liver disease with insulin resistance. Am J Med 107: 450–455
60. Assy N, Kaita K, Mymin D, Levy C, Rosser B, Minuk G (2000) Fatty infiltration of liver in hyperlipidemic patients. Dig Dis Sci 45: 1929–1934
61. Caldwell SH, Swerdlow RH, Khan EM, Iezzoni JC, Hespenheide EE, Parks JK, Parker WD (1999) Mitochondrial abnormalities in non-alcoholic steatohepatitis. J Hepatol 31: 430–434
62. Sozo A, Arrese M, Glasinovic JC (2001) Evidence of intestinal bacterial overgrowth in patients with NASH (abstract). Gastroenterology 120: 118
63. Gamez J, Ferreiro BS, Accarino ML, Guarner L, Tadesse S, Marti RA, Andreu AL, Raguer N, Cervera C, Hirano M (2002) Phenotypic variation in a Spanish family with MNGIE. Neurology 59: 455–457
64. Powell EE, Searle J, Mortimer R (1989) Steatohepatitis associated with limb lipodystrophy. Gastroenterology 97: 1022–1024
65. Feliciani C, Amerio P (1999) Madelung's disease: inherited from an ancient Mediterranean population? N Engl J Med 340: 1481
66. Wasserman JM, Thung SN, Berman R, Bodenheimer HC, Sigal SH (2001) Hepatic Weber-Christian disease. Semin Liver Dis 21: 115–118
67. Dahl MG, Gregory MM, Scheuer PJ (1971) Liver damage due to methotrexate in patients with psoriasis. BMJ 1: 625–630
68. Pirovino M, Muller O, Zysset T, Honegger U (1988) Amiodarone-induced hepatic phospholipidosis: correlation of morphological and biochemical findings in an animal model. Hepatology 8: 591–598
69. Pinto HC, Baptista A, Camilo ME, de Costa EB, Valente A, de Moura MC (1995) Tamoxifen-associated steatohepatitis—report of three cases. J Hepatol 23: 95–97
70. Cotrim HP, Andrade ZA, Parana R, Portugal M, Lyra LG, Freitas LA (1999) Nonalcoholic steatohepatitis: a toxic liver disease in industrial workers. Liver 19: 263–264
71. Chitturi S, Farrell GC (2001) Etiopathogenesis of nonalcoholic steatohepatitis. Semin Liver Dis 21: 27–41
72. Caldwell SH, Hespenheide EE (2002) Subacute liver failure in obese females. Am J Gastroenterol 97: 2058–2062
73. Caldwell SH, Oelsner DH, Iezzoni JC, Hespenheide EE, Battle EH, Driscoll CJ (1999) Cryptogenic cirrhosis: clinical characterization and risk factors for underlying disease. Hepatology 29: 664–669
74. Ratziu V, Bonyhay L, Di Martino V, Charlotte F, Cavallaro L, Sayegh-Tainturier MH, Giral P, Grimaldi A, Opolon P, Poynard T (2002) Survival, liver failure, and hepatocellular carcinoma in obesity-related cryptogenic cirrhosis. Hepatology 35: 1485–1493
75. Garcia-Monzon C, Martin-Perez E, Iacono OL, Fernandez-Bermejo M, Majano PL, Apolinario A, Larranaga E, Moreno-Otero R (2000) Characterization of pathogenic and prognostic factors of nonalcoholic steatohepatitis associated with obesity. J Hepatol 33: 716–724

76. Mathieson UL, Franzen LE, Fryden A, Foberg U, Bodemar G (1999) The clinical significance of slightly to moderately elevated liver transaminase values in asymptomatic patients. Scand J Gastroenterol 34: 85–91
77. Patt CH, Yoo HY, Dibadj K, Flynn J, Thuluvath PJ (2003) Prevalence of transaminase abnormalities in asymptomatic, healthy subjects participating in an executive health-screening program. Digestive Diseases & Sciences 48(4): 797–801
78. Sorbi D, McGill DB, Thistle JL, Therneau TM, Henry J, Lindor KD (2000) An assessment of the role of liver biopsies in asymptomatic patients with chronic liver test abnormalities. Am J Gastroenterol 95: 3206–3210
79. Hay JE, Czaja AJ, Rakela J, Ludwig J (1989) The nature of unexplained chronic aminotransferase elevations of a mild to moderate degree in asymptomatic patients. Hepatology 9: 193–197
80. Daniel S, Ben-Menachem T, Vasudevan G, Ma CK, Blumenkehl M (1999) Prospective evaluation of unexplained chronic liver transaminase abnormalities in asymptomatic and symptomatic patients. Am J Gastroenterol 94: 3010–3014
81. Caldwell SH, Hespenheide EE, Redick JA, Iezzoni JC, Battle EH, Sheppard BL (2001) A pilot study of a thiazolidinedione, troglitazone, in nonalcoholic steatohepatitis. Am J Gastroenterol 96: 519–525
82. Mofrad P, Contos MJ, Haque M, Sargeant C, Fisher RA, Luketic VA, Sterling RK, Shiffman ML, Stravitz RT, Sanyal AJ (2003) Clinical and histologic spectrum of NAFLD associated with normal ALT values. Hepatology 37: 1286–1292
83. Prati D, Taioli E, Zanella A, Della Torre E, Butelli S, Del Vecchio E, Vianello L, Zanuso F, Mozzi F, Milani S, Conte D, Colombo M, Sirchia G (2002) Updated definitions of healthy ranges for serum alanine aminotransferase levels. Ann Intern Med 137: 1–10
84. Shan Y, Bigelow C, Bonkovsky HL (2002) Prevalence of liver disease in the US population and association with iron homeostasis: analysis of data from NHANES III (abstract). Hepatology 36: 408
85. Bonkovsky H, Jawaid Q, Tortorelli K, LeClair P, Cobb J, Lambrecht R, Banner B (1999) Non-alcoholic steatohepatitis and iron: increased prevalence of mutations of the HFE gene in non-alcoholic steatohepatitis. J Hepatol 31: 421–429
86. George D, Goldwurm S, MacDonald G, Cowley LL, Walker NI, Ward PJ, Jazwinska EC, Powell LW (1998) Increased hepatic iron concentration in nonalcoholic steatohepatitis is associated with increased fibrosis. Gastroenterology 114: 311–318
87. Angulo P, Keach JC, Batts KP, Lindor KD (1999) Independent predictors of liver fibrosis in patients with nonalcoholic steatohepatitis. Hepatology 30: 1356–1362
88. Younossi ZM, Gramlich T, Bacon BR, Matteoni CA, Boparai N, O'Neill R, McCullough AJ (1999) Hepatic iron and nonalcoholic fatty liver disease. Hepatology 30: 847–850
89. Tumiel M, Whitcomb BJ, Krawitt EL (1994) Circulating antinuclear antibodies in patients with nonalcoholic steatohepatitis (abstract). Hepatology 20: 409
90. Tajiri K, Takenawa H, Yamaoka K (1997) Nonalcoholic steatohepatitis masquerading as autoimmune hepatitis. J Clin Gastrroenterol 25: 538–540
91. Nagore N, Scheuer PJ (1988) Does a linear pattern of sinusoidal IgA deposition distinguish between alcoholic and diabetic liver disease? Liver 8: 281–286
92. Caldwell SH, Hespenheide EE (2001) Obesity and cryptogenic cirrhosis. In: Leuschner U, James O, Dancygier H (eds) Steatohepatitis (ASH and NASH). Falk Symposium 121. Kluwer Academic, Norwell, MA, p 151
93. Kanjii K, Jakate S, Keshavarzian A, Jensen DM, Cotler SJ (2003) Prevalence and clinical features of associated autoantibodies in NASH. Hepatology 34: 506A
94. Rosado-Carrion B, Lindor K, Talwalker J, Miles J, Rizza R, Gorman B, Charlton M (2003) Continuous glucose monitoring and metabolic evidence of subclinical glucose intolerance in NAFLD: looking beyond the tip of the insulin resistance iceberg. Hepatology 34: 508A
95. Adams LA, Keach J, Lindor KD, Angulo P (2003) Lipid profiles in NAFLD. Hepatology 34: 512A

96. Angulo P, Keach JC, Batts KP, Lindor KD (1999) Independent predictors of liver fibrosis in patients with nonalcoholic steatohepatitis. Hepatology 30: 1356–1362
97. Nanji AA, French SW, Freeman JB (1986) Serum alanine aminotransferase to aspartate aminotransferase ratio and degree of fatty liver in morbidly obese patients. Enzyme 36: 266–269
98. Sorbi D, McGill DB, Thistle JL, Therneau TM, Henry J, Lindor KD (2000) An assessment of the role of liver biopsies in asymptomatic patients with chronic liver test abnormalities. Am J Gastroenterol 95: 3206–3210
99. Garcia-Monzon C, Martin-Perez E, Iacono OL, Fernandez-Bermejo M, Majano PL, Apolinario A, Larranaga E, Moreno-Otero R (2000) Characterization of pathogenic and prognostic factors of nonalcoholic steatohepatitis associated with obesity. J Hepatol 33: 716–724
100. Struben VMD, Hespenheide EE, Caldwell SH (2000) Familial patterns of nonalcoholic steatohepatitis and cryptogenic cirrhosis. Am J Med 108: 9–13
101. Dixon JB, Bathal PS, O'Brien PE (2001) Nonalcoholic fatty liver disease: predictors of nonalcoholic steatohepatitis and liver fibrosis in the severely obese. Gastroenterology 121: 91–100
102. Harrison SA, Hayashi P (2002) Clinical factors associated with fibrosis in 102 patients with non-alcoholic steatohepatitis (abstract). Hepatology 36: 412
103. Costanzo M, Miele L, Di Rocco P, Forgione A, Alfei B, Pompili M, Rapacini GL, Grieco A, Gasbarrini G (2002) Serum markers of fibrogenesis and fibrosis in nonalcoholic steatohepatitis (abstract). Hepatology 36: 412
104. Iijima H, Moriyasu F, Tsuchiya K, Sasaki S, Suzuki S (2003) Diagnosis of NASH using Kupffer imaging of contrast enhanced ultrasound. Hepatology 34: 514A
105. Ratziu V, Le Calvez S, Imber-Bismut F, Messous D, Charlotte F, Bonyhay L, Munteanu M, Poynard T (2003) Diagnostic value of biochemical markers (Fibrotest) for the prediction of liver fibrosis in patients with NAFLD. Hepatology 34: 510A
106. Merriman RB, Ferrell LD, Patti MG, Ostroff JW, Bagetelos K, Aouizerat BE, Bass NB (2003) Histologic correlation of paired right and left lobe biopsies in morbidly obese individuals with suspected NAFLD. Hepatology 34: 232A
107. Ewe K (1981) Bleeding after liver biopsy does not correlate with indices of peripheral coagulation. Dig Dis Sci 26: 388–393
108. Piccinino F, Sagnelli E, Pasquale G, Giusti G (1986) Complication following percutaneous liver biopsy. A multicenter retrospective study on 68 276 biopsies. J Hepatol 2: 165–173
109. Caldwell SH (2001) Controlling pain in liver biopsy. Am J Gastroenterol 96: 1327–1329
110. Janes CH, Lindor KD (1993) Outcome of patients hospitalized for complications after outpatient liver biopsy. Ann Intern Med 118: 96–98
111. Byron D, Minuk GY (1996) Profile of an urban hospital-based practice. Hepatology 24: 813–815
112. Mathieson UL, Franzen LE, Fryden A, Foberg U, Bodemar G (1999) The clinical significance of slightly to moderately elevated liver transaminase values in asymptomatic patients. Scand J Gastroenterol 34: 85–91
113. Matteoni CA, Younossi ZM, Gramlich T, Boparai N, Liu YC, McCullough AJ (1999) Nonalcoholic fatty liver disease: a spectrum of clinical and pathological severity. Gastroenterology 116: 1413–1419
114. Saadeh S, Younossi ZM, Remer EM, Gramlish T, Ong JP, Hurley M, Mullen KD, Cooper JN, Sheridan MJ (2002) The utility of radiological imaging in nonalcoholic fatty liver disease. Gastroenterology 123: 745–750
115. Hilden M, Juhl E, Thomsen AC, Christoffersen P (1973) Fatty liver persisting for up to 33 years. Acta Med Scand 194: 485–489
116. Teli MR, James OFW, Burt AD, Bennett MK, Day CP (1995) The natural history of nonalcoholic fatty liver: a followup study. Hepatology 22: 1714–1719

117. Lee RG (1989) Nonalcoholic steatohepatitis: a study of 49 patients. Hum Pathol 20: 594–598
118. Powell EE, Cooksley WG, Hanson R, Searll J, Halliday JW, Powell LW (1990) The natural history of nonalcoholic steatohepatitis: a follow-up study of 42 patients for up to 21 years. Hepatology 11: 74–80
119. Bacon BR, Farahvish MJ, Janney CG, Neuschwander-Tetri BA (1994) Non-alcoholic steatohepatitis: an expanded clinical entity. Gastroenterology 107: 1103–1109
120. Ratziu V, Giral P, Charlotte F, Bruckert E, Thibault V, Theodorou I et al (2000) Liver fibrosis in overweight patients. Gastroenterology 118: 1117–1123
121. Harrison SA, Torgerson S, Hayashi PH (2003) The natural history of NAFLD: a clinical histopathological study. Am J Gastroenterol 98: 2042–2047
122. Gaede P, Vedel P, Larsen N, Jenesn GVH, Parving H-H, Pendersen O (2003) Multifactorial intervention and cardiovascular disease in patients with type 2 diabetes. N Engl J Med 348: 383–393
123. Ioannou GN, Weiss NS, Kowdley KV, Dominitz JA (2003) Is obesity a risk factor for cirrhosis-related death or hospitalization? A population based cohort study. Gastroenterology 125: 1053–1059
124. Sasaki A, Horiuchi N, Hasegawa K, Uehara M (1989) Mortality and causes of death in type 2 diabetic patients. Diabetes Res Clin Pract 7: 33–40
125. Caldwell SH, Han K, Hess CE (1997) Thrombocytopenia and unrecognized cirrhosis. Ann Intern Med 127: 572–573
126. Sozo A, Arrese M, Glasinovic JC (2001) Evidence of intestinal bacterial overgrowth in patients with NASH. Gastroenterology 120: A-118
127. Caldwell SH, Swerdlow RH, Khan EM, Iezzoni JC, Hespenheide EE, Parks JK, Parker WD (1999) Mitochondrial abnormalities in non-alcoholic steatohepatitis. J Hepatol 31: 430–434
128. Sanyal AJ, Campbell-Sargent C, Mirshahi F, Rizzo WB, Contos MJ, Sterling RK, Luketic VA, Shiffman ML, Clore JN (2001) Nonalcoholic steatohepatitis: association of insulin resistance and mitochondrial abnormalities. Gastroenterology 120: 1183–1192
129. Johns DR (1995) Mitochondrial DNA and disease. N Engl J Med 333: 638–644
130. Al-Osaimi A, Berg CL, Caldwell SH (2002) Intermittent disconjugate gaze: a novel finding in NASH and cryptogenic cirrhosis (abstract). Hepatology 36: 408A
131. Sanyal AJ, Contos MJ, Sterling RK, Luketic VA, Shiffman ML, Stravitz RT, Mills AS (2003) Nonalcoholic fatty liver disease in patients with hepatitis C is associated with features of the metabolic syndrome. Am J Gastroenterol 98: 2064–2071
132. Ayata G, Gordon FD, Lewis WD, Pomfret E, Pomposelli JJ, Jenkins RL, Khettry U (2002) Cryptogenic cirrhosis: clinicopathologic findings at and after liver transplantation. Hum Pathol 33: 1098–1104
133. Powell EE, Cooksley WG, Hanson R, Searll J, Halliday JW, Powell LW (1990) The natural history of nonalcoholic steatohepatitis: a follow-up study of 42 patients for up to 21 years. Hepatology 11: 74–80
134. Nosadini R, Avogaro A, Mollo F, Marescotti C, Tiengo A, Duner E, Merkel C, Gatta A, Zuin R, de Kreutzenberg S et al (1984) Carbohydrate and lipid metabolism in cirrhosis. Evidence that hepatic uptake of gluconeogenic precursors and of free fatty acids depends on effective hepatic flow. J Clin Endocrinol Metab 58: 1125–1132
135. Contos MJ, Cales W, Sterling RK, Lukeric VA, Shiffman ML, Mills AS, Fisher RA, Ham J, Sanyal AJ (2001) Development of nonalcoholic fatty liver disease after orthotopic liver transplantation for cryptogenic cirrhosis. Liver Transpl 7: 363–373
136. Struben VMD, Hespenheide EE, Caldwell SH (2000) Familial patterns of nonalcoholic steatohepatitis (NASH) and cryptogenic cirrhosis. Am J Med 108: 9–13
137. Willner IR, Waters B, Patil SR, Reuben A, Morelli J, Riely CA (2001) Ninety patients with nonalcoholic steatohepatitis: insulin resistance, familial tendency and severity of disease. American Journal of Gastroenterology 96(10): 2957–2961

138. Nagore N, Scheuer PJ (1988) Does a linear pattern of sinusoidal IgA deposition distinguish between alcoholic and diabetic liver disease. Liver 8: 281–286
139. Poonawala A, Nair SP, Thuluvath PJ (2000) Prevalence of obesity and diabetes in patients with cryptogenic cirrhosis: a case-control study. Hepatology 32: 689–692
140. Ong J, Younossi ZM, Reddy V, Price LL, Gramlich T, Mayes J, Boparis N (2001) Cryptogenic cirrhosis and post-transplantation non-alcoholic fatty liver disease. Liver Transplantation 7: 797–801
141. Nair S, Mason A, Eason J, Loss G, Perillo RP (2002) Is obesity an independent risk factor for hepatocellular carcinoma in cirrhosis? Hepatology 36: 150–155
142. Ratziu V, Bonyhay L, Di Martino V, Charlotte F, Cavallaro L, Sayegh-Tainturier MH, Giral P, Grimaldi A, Opolon P, Poynard T (2002) Survival, liver failure, and hepatocellular carcinoma in obesity-related cryptogenic cirrhosis. Hepatology 35: 1485–1493
143. Wanless IR, Wong F, Blendis LM, Greig P, Heathcote EJ, Levy G (1995) Hepatic and portal vein thrombosis in cirrhosis: possible role in the development of parenchymal extinction and portal hypertension. Hepatology 21(5): 1238–1247
144. El-Serag H, Davila JA, Petersen NJ, McGlynn KA (2003) The continuing increase in the incidence of hepatocellular carcinoma in the US: an update. Ann Intern Med 139: 817–823
145. Ong JP, Younossi ZM (2002) Is hepatocellular carcinoma part of the natural history of nonalcoholic steatohepatitis? Gastroenterology 123: 375–378
146. Murphy TK, Calle EE, Rodriquez C, Khan HS, Thun MJ (2000) Body mass index and colon cancer mortality in a large prospective study. Am J Epidemiol 152: 847–854
147. Yang S, Lin HZ, Hwang J, Chacko VP, Diehl AM (2001) Hepatocyte hyperplasia in noncirrhotic fatty livers: is obesity-related hepatic steatosis a premalignant condition? Cancer Res 61: 5016–5023
148. El-Sarag HB, Richardson PA, Everhart JE (2001) The role of diabetes in hepatocellular carcinoma: a case control study among United States veterans. Am J Gastroenterol 96: 2462–2467
149. Cotrim HP, Parana R, Braga E, Lyra L (2000) Nonalcoholic steatohepatitis and hepatocellular carcinoma: natural history? Am J Gastroenterol 95: 3018–3019
150. Zen Y, Katayanagi K, Tsuneyama K, Harada K, Araki I, Nakanuma Y (2001) Hepatocellular carcinoma arising in non-alcoholic steatohepatitis. Pathol Int 51: 127–131
151. Bugianesi E, Leone N, Vanni E, Marchesini G, Brunello F, Carucci P, Musso A, de Paolis P, Capussotti L, Salizzoni M, Rizzetto M (2002) Expanding the natural history of nonalcoholic steatohepatitis from cryptogenic cirrhosis to hepatocellular carcinoma. Gastroenterology 123: 134–140
152. Marrero JA, Fontana RJ, Su GL, Conjeevarum HS, Emick DM, Lok AS (2002) NAFLD may be a common underlying liver disease in patients with hepatocellular carcinoma in the US. Hepatology 36: 1349–1354
153. Day CP, James OFW (1998) Steatohepatitis: A tale of two hits. Gastroenterology 114: 842–845
154. DiMauro S, Schon EA (2003) Mitochondrial respiratory-chain diseases. N Engl J Med 348: 2656–2668
155. Carrozzo R, Hirano M, Fromenty B, Casali C, Santorelli FM, Bonilla E, DiMauro S, Schon EA, Miranda AF (1998) Multiple mtDNA deletions features in autosomal dominant and recessive diseases suggest distinct pathogeneses. Neurology 50: 99–106
156. Hoek JB, Cahill A, Pastorino JG (2002) Alcohol and mitochondria: a dysfunctional relationship. Gastroenterology 122: 2049–2063
157. Green DR, Reed JC (1998) Mitochondria and apoptosis. Science 281: 1309–1312
158. Caldwell SH, Chang C (2004) Mitochondria in NAFL. Clin Liver Dis Ed. AJ Sanyal, in press

159. Bereiter-Hahn J, Voth M (1994) Dynamics of mitochondria in living cells: shape changes, dislocations, fusion and fission of mitochondria. Microsc Res Tech 27: 198–219
160. Hepatocyte Ultrastructure Text—University of Virginia library
161. Kuroiwa T, Ohta T, Kuroiwa H, Shigeyuki K (1994) Molecular and cellular mechanisms of mitochondrial nuclear division and mitochondriokinesis. Microsc Res Tech 27: 220–232
162. Lea PJ, Temkin RJ, Freeman KB, Mitchell GA, Robinson BH (1994) Variations in mitochondrial ultrastructure and dynamics observed by high resolution scanning electron microscopy (HRSEM). Microsc Res Tech 27: 269–277
163. Lehmann TG, Wheeler MD, Schwabe RF, Connor HD, Schoonhoven R, Bunzendahl H, Samulski RJ, Thurman RG (2000) Gene delivery of Cu/Zn-superoxide dismutase improves graft function after transplantation of fatty livers in the rat. Hepatology 32: 1255–1264
164. Dianzani MU (1954) Uncoupling of oxidative phosphorylation in mitochondria from fatty livers. Biochim Biophys Acta 14: 514–532
165. Dianzani MU (1957) The content of adenosine polyphosphates in fatty livers. Biochem J 65: 116–124
166. Sternlieb I (1968) Mitochondrial and fatty changes in hepatocytes of patients with Wilson's disease. Gastroenterology 55: 354-362
167. Chedid A, Mendenhall CL, Tosch T, Chen T, Rabin L, Garcia-Pont P, Goldberg SJ, Kiernan T, Seeff LB, Sorrell M et al (1986) Significance of megamitochondria in alcoholic liver disease. Gastroenterology 90: 1858–1864
168. Caldwell SH, Swerdlow RH, Khan EM, Iezzoni JC, Hespenheide EE, Parks JK, Parker WD Jr. (1999) Mitochondrial abnormalities in NASH. J Hepatol 31: 430–434
169. Sanyal AJ, Campbell-Sargent C, Mirshani F, Rizzo WB, Contos MJ, Sterling RK, Luketic VA, Shiffman ML, Clore JN (2001) Nonalcoholic steatohepatitis: association of insulin resistance and mitochondrial abnormalities. Gastroenterology 120: 1183–1192
170. Sternlieb I, Berger JE (1969) Optical diffraction studies of crystalline structures in electron micrographs. J Cell Biol 43: 448–455
171. Caldwell SH, Hespenheide EE, Redick JA, Iezzoni JC, Battle EH, Sheppard BL (2001) A pilot study of a thiazolidinedione, troglitazone, in nonalcoholic steatohepatitis. Am J Gastroenterol 96: 519–525
172. Williams WP, Selstam E, Brain T (1998) X-ray diffraction studies of the structural organization of prolamellar bodies isolated from Zea mays. FEBS Lett 422: 252–254
173. Deng Y, Kohlwein SD, Manella CA (2002) Fasting induces cyanide-resistant respiration and oxidative stress in the amoeba *Chaos carolinensis*: implications for the cubic structural transition in mitochondrial membranes. Protoplasm 219: 160–167
174. Spycher MA, Ruttner JR (1968) Kristalloide Einschlusse in menschlichen Lebermitochondrien. Virchows Arch B Cell Pathol 1: 211–221
175. Wolf SG, Frenkiel D, Arad T, Finkel SE, Kolter R, Minsky A (1999) DNA protection by stress-induced biocrystallization. Nature 400: 83–85
176. Le TH, Caldwell SH, Redick JA, Sheppard BL, Davis CA, Arseneau KO, Iezzoni JC, Hespenheide EE, Peterson T (2004) The lobular distribution of megamitochondria with crystalline inclusions in type 3–4 NAFL
177. Dianzani MU, Scuro S (1956) The effects of some inhibitors of oxidative phosphorylation on the morphology and enzymatic activities of mitochondria. Biochem J 62: 205–215
178. Vendemiale G, Grattagliano I, Caraceni P, Caraccio G, Domenicali M, Dall'Agata M, Trevisani F, Guerrieri F, Bernardi M, Altomare E (2001) Mitochondrial oxidative injury and energy metabolism alteration in rat fatty liver: effect of the nutritional status. Hepatology 33: 808–815
179. Junnila M, Rahko T, Sukura A, Lindberg LA (2000) Reduction of carbon tetrachloride induced hepatotoxic effects by oral administration of betaine in male Han-Wistar rats: a morphometric histologic study. Vet Med 37: 231–238

180. Lehmann TG, Wheeler MD, Schwabe RF, Connor HD, Schoonhoven R, Bunzendahl H, Brenner DA, Jude Samulski R, Zhong Z, Thurman RG (2000) Gene delivery of Cu/Zn-superoxide dismutase improves graft function after transplantation of fatty liver in the rat. Hepatology 32: 1255–1264
181. Trevasani F, Colantoni A, Caraceni P, Van Thiel DH (1996) The use of donor fatty livers for liver transplantation: a challenge or a quagmire. J Hepatol 22: 114–121
182. Perez-Carreras M, Del Hoyo P, Martin MA, Rubio JC, Martin A, Castellano G, Colina F, Arenas J, Solis-Herruzo JA (2003) Defective hepatic mitochondrial respiratory chain in patients with nonalcoholic steatohepatitis. Hepatology 38(4): 999–1007
183. Cortez-Pinto H, Chatham J, Chako VP, Arnold C, Rasid A, Diehl AM (1999) Alterations in liver ATP homeostasis in human nonalcoholic steatohepatitis: a pilot study. JAMA 282: 1659–1664
184. Chavin KD, Yang SQ, Lin HZ, Chatham J, Chakko VP, Hoek JB, Walajtys-Rode E, Rashid A, Chen CH, Huang CC, Wu TC, Lane MD, Diehl AM (1999) Obesity induces expression of uncoupling protein-2 in hepatocytes and promotes liver ATP depletion. J Biol Chem 274: 5692–5700
185. Diehl AM, Hoek JB (1999) Mitochondrial uncoupling: role of uncoupling protein anion carriers and relationship to thermogenesis and weight control, 'the benefits of losing control'. J Bioenerg Biomembr 31: 493–506
186. Baffy G, Zhang CY, Glickman JN, Lowell BB (2002) Obesity-related fatty liver is unchanged in mice deficient for mitochondrial UCP-2. Hepatology 35: 753–761
187. Pessayre D, Mansouri A, Fromenty B (2002) Nonalcoholic steatosis and steatohepatitis V. Mitochondrial dysfunction in steatohepatitis. Am J Physiol Gastrointest Liver Physiol 282: G193–G199
188. Caldwell S, Chang C, Redick J, Davis C, Krugner-Higby L, Al-Osaimi A (2004) The ballooned hepatocyte in NAFL: degenerative or adaptive? Submitted to EASL
189. Ikura Y, Ohsasa M, Ogawa Y, Kaneda K, Hai E, Kayo S, Yoshima N, Shirai N, Sugama Y, Fujino H, Itabe H, Ueda M (2003) Localization of oxidized phosphatidylcholine in steatotic livers: its relation to oxidative injury in fatty liver disorders. Hepatology 34: 507A
190. Fournier E, Peresson R, Guy G, Hermier D (1997) Relationship between storage and secretion of hepatic lipids in two breeds of geese with different susceptibility to liver steatosis. Poultry Sci 76: 599–607
191. Krugner-Higby L, Attie A, Schueler K, Thuren T, Shelness G, Wendland A. Hyperlipidemia in California mice (*Peromyscus californicus*) due to increased hepatic secretion of VLDL
192. Silva JE (2003) The thermogenic effect of thyroid hormone and its clinical implications. Ann Intern Med 139: 205–213
193. Dulloo AG (2002) A sympathetic defense against obesity. Science 297: 780–781
194. Bachman ES, Dhillon H, Zhang CY, Cinti S, Bianco AC, Kobilka BK, Lowell BB (2002) betaAR signaling required for diet-induced thermogenesis and obesity resistance. Science 297: 843–845
195. Li Z, Oben JA, Yang S, Lin H, Diehl AM (2003) Norepinephrin mediates effects of leptin deficiency on hepatic innate immune system in a mouse model of NASH. Hepatology 34: 192A
196. Struben VMD, Hespenheide EE, Caldwell SH (2000) Familial patterns of nonalcoholic steatohepatitis (NASH) and cryptogenic cirrhosis. Am J Med 108: 9–13
197. Willner IR, Waters B, Patil SR, Reuben A, Morelli J, Riely CA (2001) Ninety patients with nonalcoholic steatohepatitis: insulin resistance, familial tendency and severity of disease. Am J Gastroenterol 96: 2957–2961
198. Caldwell SH, Harris DM, Patrie J, Hespenheide EE (2002) Are NASH and cryptogenic cirrhosis under diagnosed in African Americans? Am J Gastroenterol 97: 1496–1500
199. Schapira AHV (1997) Mitochondrial disorders: an overview. J Bioenerg Biomembr 29: 105–107

200. Schon EA, Bonilla E, DiMauro S (1997) Mitochondrial DNA mutations and pathogenesis. J Bioenerg Biomembr 29: 131–149
201. Johns DR (1995) Mitochondrial DNA and disease. N Engl J Med 333: 638–644
202. Wallace DC (1999) Mitochondrial diseases in mouse and man. Science 283: 1482–1488
203. Bohan A, Droogan O, Nolan N, Mayne P, Bonham J, Thornton P, Farrell MA, Hegarty JE (2000) Mitochondrial DNA abnormalities without significant deficiency of intramitochondrial fatty acid beta oxidation enzymes in a well defined subgroup of patients with nonalcoholic steatohepatitis (abstract). Hepatology 32: 387A
204. Carrozzo R, Hirano M, Fromenty B, Casali C, Santorelli FM, Bonilla E, DiMauro S, Schon EA, Miranda AF (1998) Multiple mtDNA deletions features in autosomal dominant and recessive diseases suggest distinct pathogeneses. Neurology 50: 99–106
205. Hinokio Y, Suzuki S, Komatu K, Ohtomo M, Onoda M, Matsumoto M, Hirai S, Sato Y, Akai H, Ae K, Miyabayasi S, Abe R, Toyota T (1995) A new mitochondrial DNA deletion associated with diabetic amyotrophy, diabetic myoatrophy, and diabetic fatty liver. Muscle Nerve 3: S142–149
206. Feliciani C, Amerio P (1999) Madelung's disease: inherited from an ancient Mediterranean population? N Engl J Medicine 340: 1481
207. Vila MR, Gamez J, Solano A, Playan A, Schwartz S, Santorelli FM, Cervera C, Casali C, Montoya J, Villarroya F (2000) Uncoupling protein-1 m RNA expression in lipomas from patients bearing pathogenic mitochondrial DNA mutations. Biochem Biophys Res Commun 278: 800–802
208. Guillausseau PJ, Massin P, Dubois-LaForgue D, Timsit J, Virally M, Gin H, Bertin E, Blickle JF, Bouhanick B, Cahen J, Caillat-Zucman S, Charpentier G, Chedin P, Derrien C, Ducluzeau PH, Grimaldi A, Guerci B, Kaloustian E, Murat A, Olivier F, Paques M, Paquis-Flucklinger V, Porokhov B, Samuel-Lajeunesse J, Vialettes B (2001) Maternally inherited diabetes and deafness: a multicenter study. Ann Intern Med 134: 721–728
209. Kadowaki H, Tobe K, Mori Y, Sakura H, Sakuta R, Nonaka I, Hagura R, Yazaki Y, Akanuma Y, Kadowaki T (1993) Lancet 341: 893–894
210. Minana JB, Gomez-Cambronero L, Lloret A, Pallardo FV, Del Olmo J, Escudero A, Rodrigo JM, Pelliin A, Vina JR, Vina J, Sastre J (2002) Mitochondrial oxidative stress and CD95 ligand: a dual mechanism for hepatocyte apoptosis in chronic alcoholism. Hepatology 35: 1205–1214
211. Feldman G, Haouzi D, Moreau A, Durang-Schneider A-M, Bringuier A, Berson A, Mansouri A, Fau D, Pessayre D (2000) Opening of the mitochondrial permeability transition pore causes matrix expansion and outer membrane rupture in FAS-mediated hepatic apoptosis in mice. Hepatology 31: 674–683
212. Feldsteine A, Canbay A, Angulo P, Taniai M, Burgart LJ, Lindor KD (2003) Hepatocyte apoptosis in patients with non-alcoholic steatohepatitis. Quantification and clinical relevance. Gastroenterology 124: 703A
213. Rashid A, Wu T-C, Huang CC, Chen CH, Lin HZ, Yang SQ, Lee FY, Diehl AM (1999) Mitochondrial proteins that regulate apoptosis and necrosis are induced in mouse fatty liver. Hepatology 29: 1131–1138
214. Powell EE, Searle J, Mortimer R (1989) Steatohepatitis associated with limb lipodystrophy. Gastroenterology 97: 1022–1024
215. Degoul F, Sutton A, Mansouri A, Cepanec C, Degott C, Fromenty B, Beaugrand M, Valla D, Pessayre D (1995) Homozygosity for alanine in the mitochondrial targeting sequence of manganese superoxide dismutase and risk for severe alcoholic liver disease. Gastroenterology 108: 193–200
216. Petersen KF, Befroy D, Dufour S, Dziura J, Ariyan C, Rothman DL, DiPietro L, Cline GW, Shulman GI (2003) Mitochondrial dysfunction in the elderly: possible role in insulin resistance. Science 300: 1140–1142

217. Borkman M, Storlien LH, Pan DA, Jenkins AB, Chisholm DJ, Campbell LV (1993) The relationship between insulin sensitivity and the fatty-acid composition of skeletal muscle phospholipids. N Engl J Med 328: 238–244
218. Sreekumar R, Rosado B, Rasmussen D, Charlton M (2003) Hepatic gene expression in histologically progressive nonalcoholic steatohepatitis. Hepatology 38: 244–251
219. Angulo P (2002) Nonalcoholic fatty liver disease. N Engl J Med 346: 1221–1231
220. Tokar JL, Berg CL (2002) Therapeutic options in nonalcoholic fatty liver disease. Curr Treat Opt Gastroenterol 5: 425–436
221. Agrawal S, Bonkovsky HL (2002) Management of nonalcoholic steatohepatitis. J Clin Gastroenterol 35: 253–261
222. Younossi ZM, Diehl AM, Ong J (2002) Nonalcoholic fatty liver disease: an agenda for clinical research. Hepatology 35: 746–752
223. McCullough AJ (2002) Update on nonalcoholic fatty liver disease. J Clin Gastroenterol 34: 255–262
224. Davies MJ, Baer DJ, Judd JT, Brown ED, Campbell WS, Taylor PR (2003) Effects of moderate alcohol intake on fasting insulin and glucose concentrations and insulin sensitivity in postmenopausal women. JAMA 287: 2559–2562
225. Dixon JB, Bathal PS, O'Brien PE (2001) Nonalcoholic fatty liver disease: predictors of nonalcoholic steatohepatitis and liver fibrosis in the severely obese. Gastroenterology 121: 91–100
226. Cotrim HP, Andrade ZA, Parana R, Portugal M, Lyra LG, Freitas LA (1999) Nonalcoholic steatohepatitis: a toxic liver disease in industrial workers. Liver 19: 263–264
227. Brodkin CA, Daniell W, Checkoway H, Echeverria D, Johnson J, Wang K, Sohaey R, Green D, Redlich C, Gretch D, Rosenstock L (1995) Hepatic ultrasonic changes in workers exposed to perchloroethylene. Occup Environ Med 52: 679–685
228. Redlich CA, Cullen MR (1997) Nonalcoholic steatohepatitis (letter). Ann Intern Med 127: 410
229. Saksena S, Johnson J, Ouiff SP, Elias E (1999) Diet and exercise: important first steps in therapy of NASH (abstract). Hepatology 30: 436
230. Bertram SR, Venter I, Stewart RI (1990) Weight loss in obese women—exercise versus dietary education. S Afr Med J 78: 15–18
231. Eriksson S, Eriksson KF, Bondesson L (1986) Nonalcoholic steatohepatitis in obesity: a reversible condition. Acta Med Scand 220: 83–88
232. Ueno T, Sugawara H, Sujaku K, Hashimoto O, Tsuji R, Tamaki S, Torimura T, Inuzuka S, Sata M, Tanikawa K (1997) Therapeutic effects of restricted diet and exercise in obese patients with fatty liver. J Hepatol 27: 103–107
233. Keeffe EB, Adesman PW, Stenzel P, Palmer RM (1987) Steatosis and cirrhosis in an obese diabetic resolution of fatty liver by fasting. Dig Dis Sci 32: 441–445
234. Palmer M, Schaffner F (1990) Effect of weight reduction on hepatic abnormalities in overweight patients. Gastroenterology 99: 1408–1412
235. Rozental P, Biava C, Spencer H, Zimmerman HJ (1967) Liver morphology and function tests in obesity and during total starvation. Am J Dig Dis 12: 198–208
236. Drenick EJ, Simmons F, Murphy J (1970) Effect on hepatic morphology of treatment of obesity by fasting, reducing diets and small-bowel bypass. N Engl J Med 282: 829–834
237. Andersen T, Gluud C, Franzmann M-B, Christoffersen P (1991) Hepatic effects of dietary weight loss in morbidly obese subjects. J Hepatol 12: 224–229
238. Vajro P, Fontanella A, Perna C, Orso G, Tedesco M, de Vincenzo A (1994) Persistent hypertransaminasemia resolving after weight reduction in obese children. J Pediatr 125: 239–241
239. Vajro P, Franzese A, Valerio G, Iannucci MP, Aragione N (2000) Lack of efficacy of ursodeoxycholic acid for the treatment of liver abnormalities in obese children. J Pediatr 136: 739–743

240. Park HS, Kim MW, Shin ES (1995) Effect of weight control on hepatic abnormalities in obese patients with fatty liver. J Korean Med Sci 10414–10421
241. Eriksson J, Tuominen J, Valle T, Sundberg S, Sovijarvi A, Lindholm H, Tuomilehto J, Koivisto V (1998) Aerobic endurance exercise or circuit-type resistance training for individuals with impaired glucose tolerance? Horm Metab Res 30: 37–41
242. Franzese A, Vajro P, Argenziano A, Puzziello A, Iannucci MP, Saviano MC, Brunetti F, Rubino A (1997) Liver involvement in obese children: ultrasonography and liver enzyme levels at diagnosis and during follow-up in an Italian population. Dig Dis Sci 42: 1428–1432
243. Okita M, Hayashi M, Sasagawa T, Takagi K, Suzuki K, Kinoyama S, Ito T, Yamada G (2001) Effect of a moderately energy-restricted diet on obese patients with fatty liver. Nutrition 17: 542–547
244. Capron JP, Delamarre J, Dupas JL, Braillon A, Degott C, Quenum C (1982) Fasting in obesity: another cause of liver injury with alcoholic hyaline? Dig Dis Sci 54: 374–377
245. Hickman IJ, Jonsson JR, Prins JB, Ash S, Purdie DM, Clouston AD, Powell EE (2003) Benefit of sustained weight loss and exercise in overweight patients with liver disease (abstract). Hepatology 34: 504A
246. van Baak MA (1999) Exercise training and substrate utilization in obesity. Int J Obes 23 (Suppl 3): S11–S17
247. Hoppeler H (1999) Skeletal muscle substrate metabolism. Int J Obes 23 (Suppl 3): S7–S10
248. Eden KB, Orleans T, Mulrow CD, Pender NJ, Teutsch SM (2002) Does counseling by clinicians improve physical activity? A summary of the evidence for the US preventive services task force. Ann Intern Med 137: 208–215
249. Tuomilehto J, Lindstrom J, Eriksson JG, Valle TT, Hamalainen H, Ilanne-Parikka P, Keinanen-Kiukaanniemi S, Laakso M, Louheranta A, Rastas M, Salminen V, Uusitupa M (2001) Prevention of type 2 diabetes mellitus by changes in lifestyle among subjects with impaired glucose tolerance. N Engl J Med 344: 1343–1350
250. Epstein FH (2000) Exercise limitations in health and disease. N Engl J Med 343: 632–640
251. Kraus WE, Houmard JA, Duscha BD, Knetzger KJ, Wharton MB, McCartney JS, Bales CW, Henes S, Samsa GP, Otvos JD, Kulkarni KR, Slentz CA (2002) Effects of the amount and intensity of exercise on plasma lipoproteins. N Engl J Med 347: 1483–1492
252. Jackicic JM, Winters C, Lang W, Wing RR (1999) Effects of intermittent exercise and use of home exercise equipment adherence, weight loss, and fitness in overweight women: a randomized trial. JAMA 282: 1554–1560
253. Sothern MS, Loftin JM, Udall JN, Suskind RM, Ewing TL, Tang SC, Blecker U (2000) Safety, feasibility, and efficacy of a resistance training program in preadolescent obese children. Am J Med 319: 370–375
254. Schipper MEI, van Soest H, van Hattum J (2002) Improvement of steatosis after extracorporeal whole body hyperthermia in patients with chronic hepatitis C virus infection. Single Topic Conference on NASH Syllabus, Atlanta, Georgia, 2002
255. Dulloo AG (2002) Biomedicine. A sympathetic defense against obesity. Science 297: 780–781
256. Bachman ES, Dhillon H, Zhang CY, Cinti S, Bianco AC, Kobilka BK, Lowell BB (2002) betaAR signaling required for diet-induced thermogenesis and obesity resistance. Science 297: 843–845
257. Cheuvront SN (2000) The Zone diet and athletic performance. Sports Med 27: 213–228
258. Landers P, Wolfe MM, Glore S, Guild R, Phillips L (2002) Effect of weight loss plans on body composition and diet duration. J Oklah State Med Assoc 95: 329–331
259. Amir R, Solga SF, Clark JM, Torbenson M, Cohen A, Diehl AM, Magnuson TH (2003) Dietary composition and fatty liver disease. Hepatology 34: 513A

260. Anonymous. (1998) Executive summary of the clinical guidelines on the identification, evaluation, and treatment of overweight and obesity in adults. Arch Intern Med 158: 1855–1867
261. Krauss RM, Eckel RH, Howard B, Appel LJ, Daniels SR, Deckelbaum RJ, Erdman JW Jr, Kris-Etherton P, Goldberg IJ, Kotchen TA, Lichtenstein AH, Mitch WE, Mullis R, Robinson K, Wylie-Rosett J, St Jeor S, Suttie J, Tribble DL, Bazzarre TL (2000) AHA dietary guidelines: revision 2000. A statement for healthcare professionals from the nutrition committee of the American Heart Association. Stroke 31: 2751–2766
262. Clark MJ, Sterrett JJ, Carson DS (2000) Diabetes guidelines: a summary and comparison of the recommendations of the American Diabetes Association, Veterans Health Administration, and American Association of Clinical Endocrinologists. Clin Ther 22: 899–910
263. Spieth LE, Harnish JD, Lenders CM, Raezer LB, Pereira MA, Hangen SJ, Ludwig DS (2000) A low glycemic index diet in the treatment of pediatric obesity. Arch Pediatr Adolesc Med 154: 947–951
264. Vessby B (2000) Dietary fat and insulin action in humans. Br J Nutr 83 (Suppl 1): S91–S96
265. Kurihara T, Adachi Y, Yamagata M, Abe K, Akimoto M, Hashimoto H, Ishiguro H, Niimi A, Maeda A, Shigemoto M, et al (1994) Role of eicosapentanoic acid in lipid metabolism in the liver with special reference to experimental fatty liver. Clin Ther 16: 830–837
266. Nanji AA, Sadrzadeh SMH, Yang EK, Fogt F, Meydani M, Dannenberg AJ (1995) Dietary saturated fatty acids: a novel treatment for alcoholic liver disease. Gastroenterology 109: 547–554
267. Lokesh B, LiCari J, Kinsella JE (1992) Effect of different dietary triglycerides on liver fatty acids and prostaglandin synthesis by mouse peritoneal cells. J Parenter Enteral Nutr 16: 316–321
268. Lanza-Jacoby S, Smythe C, Phetteplace H, Tabares A (1992) Adaptation to a fish oil diet before inducing sepsis in rats prevents fatty infiltration of the liver. J Parenter Enteral Nutr 16: 353–358
269. Grattagliano I, Palmieri VO, Palasciano G (2002) Hepatotoxicity of polyunsaturated fatty acids in alcohol abuser. J Hepatol 37: 291–292
270. Luo J, Rizkalla SW, Boillot J, Alamowitch C, Chaib H, Bruzzo F, Desplanque N, Dalix AM, Durand G, Slama G (1996) Dietary (n-3) polyunsaturated fatty acids improve adipocyte insulin action and glucose metabolism in insulin-resistant rats: relation to membrane fatty acids. J Nutr 126: 1951–1958
271. Clarke SD, Baillie R, Jump DB, Nakamura MT (1997) Fatty acid regulation of gene expression. Its role in fuel partitioning and insulin resistance. Ann N Y Acad Sci 927: 178–187
272. Montagne O, Vedel I, Durand-Zalaski I (1999) Assessment of the impact of fibrates and diet on survival and their cost-effectiveness: evidence from randomized, controlled trials in coronary heart disease and health economics evaluations. Clin Ther 21: 2027–2035
273. Daubioul C, Rousseau N, Demeure R, Gallez B, Taper H, Declerck B, Delzenne N (2002) Dietary fructans, but not cellulose, decrease triglyceride accumulation in the liver of obese Zucker fa/fa rats. J Nutr 132: 967–973
274. Kolanowski J (1999) A risk-benefit assessment of anti-obesity drugs. Drug Safety 20: 119–131
275. Favreaux JT, Ryu ML, Braunstein G, Orshansky G, Park SS, Coody GL, Love LA, Fong T-L (2002) Severe hepatotoxicity associated with the dietary supplement LipoKinetix. Ann Intern Med 136: 590–595
276. Harrison SA, Fincke C, Helinski D, Torgerson S (2002) Orlistat treatment in obese, non-alcoholic steatohepatitis patients: a pilot study (abstract). Hepatology 36: 406

277. Yanovsky SZ, Yanovsky JA (2002) Obesity. N Engl J Med 346: 591–602
278. Mun EC, Blackburn GL, Matthews JB (2001) Current status of medical and surgical therapy for obesity. Gastroenterology 120: 669–681
279. Luyckx FH, Desaive C, Thiry A, Dewe W, Scheen AJ, Gielen JE, Lefebvre PJ (1998) Liver abnormalities in severely obese subjects: effect of drastic weight loss after gastroplasty. Int J Obes Relat Metab Disord 22: 222–226
280. Silverman EM, Sapala JA, Appelman HD (1995) Regression of hepatic steatosis in morbidly obese persons after gastric bypass. Am J Clin Pathol 104: 23–31
281. Ranlov I, Hardt F (1990) Regression of liver steatosis following gastroplasty or gastric bypass for morbid obesity. Digestion 47: 208–214
282. Busetto L, Tregnaghi A, De Marchi F, Segato G, Foletto M, Sergi G, Favretti F, Lise M, Enzi G (2002) Liver volume and visceral obesity in women with hepatic steatosis undergoing gastric banding. Obes Res 10: 408–411
283. Duchini A, Brunson ME (2001) Roux-en-Y gastric bypass for recurrent nonalcoholic steatohepatitis in liver transplant recipients with morbid obesity. Transplantation 72: 156–171
284. Ackerman NB (1979) Protein supplementation in the management of degenerating liver function after jejunoileal bypass. Surg Gynecol Obstet 149: 8–14
285. Drenick EJ, Fisler J, Johnson D (1982) Hepatic steatosis after intestinal bypass. Prevention and reversal by metronidazole, irrespective of protein-calorie malnutrition. Gastroenterology 82: 535–548
286. Laurin J, Lindor KD, Crippen JS, Gossard A, Gores GJ, Ludwig J, Rakela J, McGill DB (1996) Ursodeoxycholic acid or clofibrate in the treatment of non-alcohol-induced steatohepatitis: a pilot study. Hepatology 23: 1464–1467
287. Guma G, Viola L, Thome M, Galdame O, Albarez E (1997) Ursodeoxycholic acid in the treatment of nonalcoholic steatohepatitis: results of a prospective clinical controlled trial (abstract). Hepatology 26: 387
288. Ceriani R, Brunati S, Morini L, Sacchi E, Colombo G (1998) Effect of ursodeoxycholic acid plus diet in patients with nonalcoholic steatohepatitis (abstract). Hepatology 28: 386
289. Mendez-Sanchez N, Gonzalez V, Pichardo-Bahena R, Uribe M (2002) Weight reduction and ursodeoxycholic acid in subjects with nonalcoholic fatty liver disease: a randomized, double-blind, placebo-controlled trial (abstract). Hepatology 36: 412
290. Okan A, Astarcioglu H, Tankurt E, Sagul O, Altekin E, Astarcioglu I, Gonen O (2002) Effect of ursodeoxycholic acid on hepatic steatosis in rats. Dig Dis Sci 47: 2389–2397
291. Laurin J, Lindor KD, Crippin JS, Gossard A, Gores GJ, Ludwig J, Rakela J, McGill DB (1996) Ursodeoxcholic acid or clofibrate in the treatment of non-alcoholic steatohepatitis: A pilot study. Hepatology 23: 1464–1467
292. Lindor KD, Kowdley KV, Heathcote EJ, Harrison ME, Jorgensen R, Angulo P, Lymp JF, Burgart L, Colin P (2004) Ursodeoxycholic acid for treatment of nonalcoholic steatohepatitis: results of a randomized trial. Hepatology 39(3): 770–778
293. Kerai MD, Waterfield CJ, Kenyon SH, Asker DS, Timbrell JA (2001) The effect of taurine depletion by β-alanine treatment on the susceptibility to ethanol-induced hepatic dysfunction in rats. Alcohol Alcohol 36: 29–38
294. Kerai MD, Waterfield CJ, Kenyon SH, Asker DS, Timbrell JA (1999) Reversal of ethanol-induced hepatic steatosis and lipid peroxidation by taurine: a study in rats. Alcohol Alcohol 34: 529–541
295. Zaman N, Tam YK, Jewell LD, Coutts RT (1996) Effects of taurine supplementation in parenteral nutrition-associated hepatosteatosis and lidocaine metabolism. A study using isolated rat liver perfusion. Drug Metab Dispos Biol Fate Chem 24: 534–541
296. Kerai MD, Waterfield CJ, Kenyon SH, Asker DS, Timbrell JA (1998) Taurine: protective properties against ethanol-induced hepatic steatosis and lipid peroxidation during chronic ethanol consumption in rats. Amino Acids 15: 53–76

297. Obinata K, Maruyama T, Hayashi M, Watanabe T, Nittono H (1996) Effect of taurine on the fatty liver of children with simple obesity. Adv Exp Med Biol 403: 607–613
298. Simon JB, Scheig R, Klatskin G (1968) Protection by orotic acid against the renal necrosis and fatty liver of choline deficiency. Proc Soc Exp Biol Med 129: 874–877
299. Buchman AL, Dubin M, Jenden D, Moukarzel A, Roch MH, Rice K, Gornbein J, Ament ME, Eckhert CD (1992) Lecithin increases plasma free choline and decreases hepatic steatosis in long-term total parenteral nutrition patients. Gastroenterology 102: 1363–1370
300. Demetriou AA (1992) Lecithin increases plasma free choline and decreases hepatic steatosis in long-term total parenteral nutrition patients. J Parenter Enteral Nutr 16: 487–488
301. Antisiewicz J, Nishizawa Y, Liu X, Usukura J, Wakabayashi T (1994) Suppression of the hydrazine-induced formation of megamitochondria in the rat liver by α-tocopherol. Exp Mol Pathol 60: 173–187
302. Soltys K, Dikdan G, Koneru B (2001) Oxidative stress in fatty liver of obese Zucker rats: rapid amelioration and improved tolerance to warm ischemia with tocopherol. Hepatology 34: 13–18
303. Lavine JE (2000) Vitamin E treatment of nonalcoholic steatohepatitis in children: a pilot study. J Pediatr 136: 711–713
304. Brown BG, Zhao XQ, Chait A, Fisher LD, Cheung MC, Morse JS, Dowdy AA, Marino EK, Bolson EL, Alaupovic P, Frohlich J, Albers JJ (2001) Simvastatin and niacin, antioxidant vitamins, or the combination for the prevention of coronary disease. N Engl J Med 345: 1583–1592
305. Fu CS, Esrason K, Alshak NS, Conteas CN, Simmons VJ (1998) Dietary lecithin, antioxidant and vitamin B complex (LAB) decrease hepatic steatosis in patients with NASH (abstract). Gastroenterology 114: 1243
306. Hasegawa T, Yoneda M, Nakamura K, Makino I, Terano A (2001) Plasma transforming growth factor-β1 level and efficacy of α-tocopherol in patients with non-alcoholic steatohepatitis: a pilot study. Aliment Pharmacol Ther 15: 1667–1672
307. Harrison SA, Torgerson S, Hayashi P, Ward J, Schenker S (2003) Vitamin E and vitamin C treatment improves fibrosis in patients with NASH. Am J Gastroenterol 98: 2485–2490
308. Alvaro D, Gigliozzi A, Piat C, Carli L, Bini A, La Rosa T, Furfaro S, Capocaccia L (1995) Effect of S-adenosyl-L-methionine on ethanol cholestasis and hepatotoxicity in isolated perfused rat liver. Dig Dis Sci 40: 1592–1600
309. Lu S (1998) Methionine adenosyltransferase and liver disease: it's all about SAM. Gastroenterology 114: 403–407
310. Colell A, Garcia-Ruiz C, Morales A, Ballesta A, Ookhtens M, Rodes J, Kaplowitz N, Fernandez-Checa JC (1997) Transport of reduced glutathione in hepatic mitochondria and mitoplasts from ethanol-treated rats: effect of membrane physical properties and S-adenosyl-methionine. Hepatology 26: 699–708
311. Lieber CS (2002) *S*-Adenosyl-L-methionine and alcoholic liver disease in animal models: implications for early intervention in human beings. Alcohol 27: 173–177
312. Nakano H, Yamaguchi M, Kaneshiro Y, Yoshida K, Kigawa G, Nagasaki H, Fujiwara Y, Matsumoto F, Kitamura N, Sasaki J, Kuzume M, Takeuchi S, Kumada K (1998) *S*-Adenosyl-L-methionine attenuates ischemia-reperfusion injury of steatotic rats. Transplant Proc 30: 3735–3736
313. Avila MA, Carretero MV, Rodriguez EN, Mato JM (1998) Regulation by hypoxia of methionine adenosyltransferase activity and gene expression in rat hepatocytes. Gastroenterology 114: 364–371
314. Mazzanti R, Arcangeli A, Salvadori G, Smorlesi C, Di Perri T, Auteri A, Boggiano CA, Pippi L, Toti M, Boncompagni P, Angioli D, Caremani M, Magnolfi F, Camarri E, Motta R, Forconi A, Tommasi AC, Lomi M, Soldi A (1978) The anti-steatotic effect of sulfo-

adenosylmethionine (SAMe) in various forms of chronic hepatopathy. Multicentric research. Minerva Med 69: 3283–3292

315. Labo G, Gasbarrini GB (1975) Therapeutic action of S-adenosylmethionine in some chronic hepatopathies. Minerva Med 66: 1563–1570
316. Labo G, Gasbarrini G, Miglio F (1972) Various effects of SAM dependent transmethylations in hepatology. Minerva Med 63: 2007–2017
317. Neuschwander-Tetri BA (2001) Betaine: an old therapy for a new scourge. Am J Gastroenterol 96: 2534–2546
318. Abdelmalek MF, Angulo P, Jorgensen RA, Sylvestre PB, Lindor KD (2001) Betaine, a promising new agent for patients with nonalcoholic steatohepatitis: results of a pilot study. Am J Gastroenterol 96: 2711–2717
319. Miglio F, Rovati LC, Santoro A, Setnikar I (2000) Efficacy and safety of oral betaine glucuronate in non-alcoholic steatohepatitis. A double-blind, randomized, parallel-group, placebo-controlled prospective clinical study. Arzneimittelforschung 50: 722–727
320. Nakano H, Nagasaki H, Yoshida K, Kigawa G, Fujiwara Y, Kitamura N, Kuzume M, Takeuchi S, Sasaki J, Shimura H, Yamaguchi M, Kumada K (1998) *N*-Acetylcysteine and anti-ICAM-1 monoclonal antibody reduce ischemia-reperfusion injury of the steatotic rat liver. Transplant Proc 30: 3763
321. Nakano H, Nagasaki H, Barama A, Boudjema K, Jaeck D, Kumada K, Tatsuno M, Baek Y, Kitamura N, Suzuki T, Yamaguchi M (1997) The effect of *N*-acetylcysteine and anti-intercellular adhesion molecule-1 monoclonal antibody against ischemia-reperfusion injury of the rat steatotic liver produced by a choline-methionine-deficient diet. Hepatology 26: 670–678
322. Gulbahar O, Karasu ZA, Ersoz G, Akarca US, Musoglu A (2000) Treatment of nonalcoholic steatohepatitis with N-acetylcysteine (abstract). Gastroenterology 118: 1444
323. Venkataramanan R, Ramachandran V, Komoroski BJ, Zhang S, Schiff PL, Strom SC (2000) Milk thistle, a herbal supplement, decreases the activity of CYP3A4 and uridine diphosphoglucuronosyl transferase in human hepatocyte cultures. Drug Metab Dispos Biol Fate Chem 28: 1270–1273
324. Azuma Y, Shinohara M, Wang PL, Hidaka A, Ohura K (2001) Histamine inhibits chemotaxis, phagocytosis, superoxide anion production, and the production of TNF-α and IL-12 by macrophages via H2-receptors. Int J Immunopharmacol 1: 1867–1875
325. Villa RF, Gorini A (1997) Pharmacology of lazaroids and brain energy metabolism: a review. Pharmacol Rev 49: 99–136
326. Li Z, Yang S, Lin H, Huang J, Watkins PA, Moser AB, DeSimone C, Song X, Diehl AM (2003) Probiotics and antibodies to TNF inhibit inflammatory activity and improve nonalcoholic fatty liver disease. Hepatology 37: 343–350
327. DeFronzo RA (1999) Pharmacologic therapy for type 2 diabetes mellitus. Ann Intern Med 131: 281–303
328. Caldwell SH, Hespenheide EE, Redick JA, Iezzoni JC, Battle EH, Sheppard BL (2001) A pilot study of a thiazolidinedione, troglitazone, in nonalcoholic steatohepatitis. Am J Gastroenterol 96: 519–525
329. Katoh S, Hata S, Matsushima M, Ikemoto S, Inoue Y, Yokoyama J, Tajima N (2001) Troglitazone prevents the rise in visceral adiposity and improves fatty liver associated with sulfonylurea therapy—a randomized controlled trial. Metabolism 50: 414–417
330. Acosta RC, Molina EG, O'Brien CB, Cobo MC, Amaro R, Neff GW, Schiff ER (2001) The use of pioglitazone in nonalcoholic steatohepatitis (abstract). Gastroenterology 120: 546
331. Neuschwander-Tetri BA, Brunt EM, Bacon BR, Sponseller C, Wehmeier KR, Hampton K (2002) Histologic improvement in NASH following increased insulin sensitivity

with the PPAR-γ ligand rosiglitazone for 48 weeks (abstract). Hepatology 36: 379
332. Galli A, Crabb DW, Ceni E, Salzano R, Melo T, Svegliati-Baroni G, Ridolfi F, Trozzi L, Surrenti C, Casini A (2002) Antidiabetic thiazolidinediones inhibit collagen synthesis and hepatic stellate cell activation in vivo and in vitro. Gastroenterology 122: 1924–1940
333. Azuma T, Tomita K, Kato S, Adachi M, Inokuchi N, Kitamura N, Nishimura T, Ishii H (2002) A pilot study of a thiazolidinedione, pioglitazone, in nonalcoholic steatohepatitis (abstract). Hepatology 36: 406
334. Sanyal AJ, Contos MJ, Sargeant C, Stravitz RT, Luketic VA, Sterling RK, Shiffman ML (2002) A randomized controlled pilot study of pioglitazone and vitamin E versus vitamin E for non-alcoholic steatohepatitis (abstract). Hepatology 36: 382
335. Vamecq J, Latruffe N (1999) Medical significance of peroxisome proliferator-activated receptors. Lancet 354: 141–148
336. Ribon V, Johnson JH, Camp HS, Saltiel AR (1998) Thiazolidinediones and insulin resistance: peroxisome proliferator-activated receptor γ activation stimulates expression of the CAP gene. Proc Natl Acad Sci U S A 95: 14751–1476
337. Kelly IE, Han TS, Walsh K, Lean ME (1999) Effects of a thiazolidinedione compound on body fat and fat distribution of patients with type 2 diabetes. Diabetes Care 22: 288–293
338. Lenhard JM, Kliewer SA, Paulik MA, Plunket KD, Lehmann JM, Weiel JE (1997) Effects of troglitazone and metformin on glucose and lipid metabolism. Biochem Pharmacol 54: 801–808
339. Aubert J, Champigny O, Saint-Marc P, Negrel R, Collins S, Ricquier D, Ailhaud G (1997) Up-regulation of UCP-2 gene expression by PPAR agonists in preadipose and adipose cells. Biochem Biophys Res Commun 238: 606–611
340. Arioglu E, Duncan-Morin J, Sebring N, Rother KI, Gottlieb N, Lieberman J, Herion D, Kleiner DE, Reynolds J, Premkumar A, Sumner AE, Hoofnagle J, Reitmen ML, Taylor SI (2000) Efficacy and safety of troglitazone in the treatment of lipodystrophy syndromes. Ann Intern Med 133: 263–274
341. Sanyal AJ, Contos MJ, Sargeant C, Stravitz RT, Luketic VA, Sterling RK, Shiffman ML (2002) A randomized controlled pilot study of pioglitazone and vitamin E versus vitamin E for non-alcoholic steatohepatitis. Hepatology 36: 382
342. Neuschwander-Tetri BA, Brunt EM, Wehmier KR, Sponseller CA, Hampton K, Bacon BR (2003) Interim results of a pilot study demonstrating the early effects of the PPAR-gamma ligand rosiglitazone on insulin sensitivity, aminotransferases, hepatic steatosis and body weight in patients with non-alcoholic steatohepatitis (2003) Hepatology 38(4): 434–440
343. Lutchman GA, Promrat K, Soza A, Heller T, Mi L, Ghany M, Park Y, Freedman R, Yanovsky J, Kleiner D, Liang TJ, Hoofnagle J (2003) Biochemical relapse and continued weight gain in subjects with NASH after discontinuation of pioglitazone. Hepatology 34: 510A
344. Lin HZ, Yang SQ, Chuckaree C, Kuhajda F, Ronnet G, Diehl AM (2000) Metformin reverses fatty liver disease in obese leptin-deficient mice. Nat Med 6: 998–1003
345. Coyle WJ, Delaney N, Yoshihashi A, Lawson P (1999) Metformin treatment in patients with nonalcoholic steatohepatitis (abstract). Gastroenterology 116: 1198
346. Urso R, Visco-Comandini U (2002) Metformin in non-alcoholic steatohepatitis. Lancet 359: 355–356
347. Marchesini G, Brizi M, Bianchi G, Tomassetti S, Zoli M, Melchionda N (2001) Metformin in non-alcoholic steatohepatitis. Lancet 358: 893–894
348. Zhou G, Myers R, Li Y, Chen Y, Shen X, Fenyk-Melody J, Wu M, Ventre J, Doebber T, Fujii N, Musi N, Hirshman MF, Goodyear LJ, Moller DE (2001) Role of AMP-activated protein kinase in mechanism of metformin action. J Clin Invest 108: 1167–1174

349. Chiasson JL, Josse RG, Gomis R, Hanefeld M, Karasik A, Laakso M (2002) Acarbose for prevention of type 2 diabetes mellitus: the STOP-NIDDM randomized trial. Lancet 359: 2072–2077
350. Santomauro ATMG, Boden G, Sliva MER, Rocha DM, Santos RF, Ursich MJM, Strassmann PG, Wajchenberg BL (1999) Overnight lowering of free fatty acids with acipimox improves insulin resistance and glucose tolerance in obese diabetic and nondiabetic subjects. Diabetes 48: 1836–1841
351. Nestler JE, Jakubowicz DJ, Iuorno MJ (2000) Role of inositolphosphoglycan mediators of insulin action in the polycystic ovary syndrome. J Pediatr Endocrinol 13 (Suppl 5): 1295–1298
352. Laurin J, Lindor KD, Crippin JS, Gossard A, Gores GJ, Ladwig J, Rakela J, McGill DB (1996) Ursodeoxcholic acid or clofibrate in the treatment of non-alcoholic steatohepatitis: A pilot study. Hepatology 23: 1464–1467
353. Saibara T, Onishi S, Ogawa Y, Yoshida S, Enzan H (1999) Bezafibrate for tamoxiphen-induced non-alcoholic steatohepatitis. Lancet 353: 1802
354. Basaranoglu M, Acbay O, Sonsuz A (1999) A controlled trial of gemfibrozil in the treatment of patients with nonalcoholic steatohepatitis. J Hepatol 31: 384
355. Caldwell SH, Zaidman JS, Hespenheide EE (2003) The liver and statin drug therapy: uncertain navigation in the sea of risk-benefit (editorial). Pharmacoepidemiology Drug Safety 12(4): 303–306
356. Horlander JC, Kwo PY, Cummings OW, Koukoulis G (2001) Atorvastatin for the treatment of NASH (abstract). Gastroenterology 120: 544
357. Nair S, Wiseman M (2002) HMG-CoA reductase inhibitors in nonalcoholic fatty liver disease: is their potential hepatotoxicity an issue in these patients? A case control study based on histology (abstract). Hepatology 36: 409
358. Phillips PS, Haas RH, Bannykh S, Hathaway S, Gray NL, Kimura BJ, Vladutiu GD, England JD (2002) Statin-associated myopathy with normal creatine kinase levels. Ann Intern Med 137: 581–585
359. Mensenkamp AR, Havekes LM, Romijn JA, Kuipers F (2001) Hepatic steatosis and very low density lipoprotein secretion: the involvement of apolipoprotein E. J Hepatol 35: 816–822
360. Charlton M, Sreekumar R, Rasmussen D, Lindor K, Nair KS (2002) Apolipoprotein synthesis in nonalcoholic steatohepatitis. Hepatology 35: 898–904
361. Facchini FS, Hua NW, Stoohs RA (2002) Effect of iron depletion in carbohydrate-intolerant patients with clinical evidence of nonalcoholic fatty liver disease. Gastroenterology 122: 931–939
362. Pawlotsky J-M (2003) Hepatitis C virus genetic variability: pathogenic and clinical implications. Clin Liver Dis 7: 45–66
363. Adinolfi LE, Utili R, Andreana A, Tripodi M-F, Marracino M, Gambardella M, Giordano M, Ruggiero G (2001) Serum HCV RNA levels correlate with histological liver damage and concur with steatosis in progression of chronic hepatitis C. Dig Dis Sci 46: 1677–1683
364. Monto A, Alonzo J, Watson JJ, Grunfeld C, Wright TL (2002) Steatosis in chronic hepatitis C: relative contributions of obesity, diabetes mellitus, and alcohol. J Hepatol 36: 729–736
365. Mihm S, Fayyazi A, Hartmann H, Ramadori G (1997) Analysis of histopathological manifestations of chronic hepatitis C virus infection with respect to virus genotype. Hepatology 25: 735–739
366. Rubbia-Brandt L, Leandro G, Spahr L, Giostra E, Quadri R, Male PJ, Negro F (2001) Liver steatosis in chronic hepatitis C: a morphological sign suggesting infection with HCV genotype 3. Histopathology 39: 119–124
367. Adinolfi LE, Gambardella M, Andreana A, Tripodi M-F, Utili R, Ruggiero G (2001) Steatosis accelerates the progression of liver damage of chronic hepatitis C patients

and correlates with specific HCV genotype and visceral obesity. Hepatology 33: 1358–1364

368. Rubbia-Brandt L, Quadri R, Abid K, Giostra E, Male PJ, Mentha G, Spahr L, Zarski J-P, Borisch B, Hadengue A, Negro F (2000) Hepatocyte steatosis is a cytopathic effect of hepatitis C virus genotype 3. J Hepatol 33: 106–115
369. Rubbia-Brandt L, Giostra E, Mentha G, Quadri R, Negro F (2001) Expression of liver steatosis in hepatitis C virus infection and pattern of response to α-interferon. J Hepatol 35: 307
370. Mendler MH, Panesar J, Govindarajan S, Milstein S, Lindsay K (2002) Changes in fatty infiltration of the liver in patients treated for chronic hepatitis C: a viral or host effect (abstract)? Hepatology 36: 404
371. Hickman IJ, Clouston AD, Macdonald GA, Purdie DM, Prins JB, Ash S, Jonsson JR, Powell EE (2002) Effect of weight reduction on liver histology and biochemistry in patients with chronic hepatitis C. Gut 53(3): 413–419
372. Nair S, Verma S, Thuluvath PJ (2002) Obesity and its effect on survival in patients undergoing orthotopic liver transplantation in the United States. Hepatology 35: 105–109
373. Czaja AJ (1997) Recurrence of nonalcoholic steatohepatitis after liver transplantation. Liver Transpl Surg 3: 185–186
374. Molloy RM, Komorowski R, Varma RR (1997) Recurrent nonalcoholic steatohepatitis and cirrhosis after liver transplantation. Liver Transpl Surg 3: 177–178
375. Carson K, Washington MK, Treem WR, Clavien PA, Hunt CM (1997) Recurrence of nonalcoholic steatohepatitis in a liver transplant recipient. Liver Transpl Surg 3: 174–176
376. Kim WR, Poterucha JJ, Porayko MK, Dickerson ER, Steers JL, Weisner RH (1996) Recurrence of nonalcoholic steatohepatitis following liver transplantation. Transplantation 62: 1802–1805
377. Contos MJ, Cales W, Sterling RK, Luketic VA, Shiffman ML, Mills AS, Fisher RA, Ham J, Sanyal AJ (2001) Development of nonalcoholic fatty liver disease after orthotopic liver transplantation for cryptogenic cirrhosis. Liver Transplantation 7: 363–373
378. Ong J, Younossi ZM, Reddy V, Price LL, Gramlich T, Mayes J, Boparis N (2001) Cryptogenic cirrhosis and post-transplantation non-alcoholic fatty liver disease. Liver Transplantation 7: 797–801
379. Cassarino DS, Swerdlow RH, Parks JK, Parker WD, Bennett JP (1998) Cyclosporin A increases resting mitochondrial membrane potential in SY5Y cells and reverses the depressed mitochondrial membrane potential of Alzheimer's disease cybrids. Biochem Biophys Res Commun 248: 168–173

Role of Leptin in Pathogenesis of NASH

Kenichi Ikejima, Tie Lang, Shunhei Yamashina, Nobuyuki Enomoto, Yoshiyuki Takei, and Nobuhiro Sato

Summary. Increasing lines of evidence indicate that obesity is an important risk factor for the exacerbation of alcoholic liver disease (ALD) and nonalcoholic steatohepatitis (NASH). Leptin, an obese gene product, is a cytokine-type hormone mainly produced from adipose tissue. Recently, it has been demonstrated that serum leptin levels are increased in patients with alcoholic cirrhosis. In this study, therefore, we investigated the role of leptin in hepatic fibrogenesis. Activated hepatic stellate cells (HSCs) produced leptin during hepatic fibrogenesis. Xenobiotic-induced hepatic fibrogenesis was almost completely abolished in ob/ob mice and Zucker (fa/fa) rats, which are inborn leptin- and leptin receptor (Ob-R)-deficient animals, respectively. Further, leptin increased transforming growth factor (TGF)-β mRNA in isolated sinusoidal endothelial cells and Kupffer cells. Moreover, leptin augmented platelet-derived growth factor (PDGF)-dependent proliferation of HSCs. Taken together, these findings lead to the postulation that leptin acts as a profibrogenic cytokine in the sinusoidal microenvironment. In conclusion, leptin most likely plays a pivotal role in the progression of hepatic fibrosis in a variety of chronic liver diseases, including NASH.

Key words. NASH, Hepatic fibrogenesis, Leptin, Sinusoidal cells, TGF-β

Introduction

Accumulating lines of evidence suggest that alcoholic liver disease (ALD) and nonalcoholic steatohepatitis (NASH) share a common pathophysiological basis, in terms of inflammation and fibrogenesis. Because NASH is often associated with metabolic syndrome, comprising obesity, type-2 diabetes, and hypertension, it is hypothesized that adipocytokines, insulin resistance, and autonomic nervous regulation play causative roles in the disease progression of NASH. Leptin, an obese gene product mainly produced from adipocytes, is a cytokine-type hormone that regulates food intake and fat metabolism through actions on the central nervous system [1]. Recently, McCullough et al. [2] reported that serum leptin levels were increased in patients with alcoholic cirrhosis. Further, hepatic stellate cells (HSCs) have been shown to produce leptin when they become activated [3]. Moreover, the coadministration of recombinant

---

Department of Gastroenterology, Juntendo University School of Medicine, 2-1-1 Hongo, Bunkyo-ku, Tokyo 113-8421, Japan

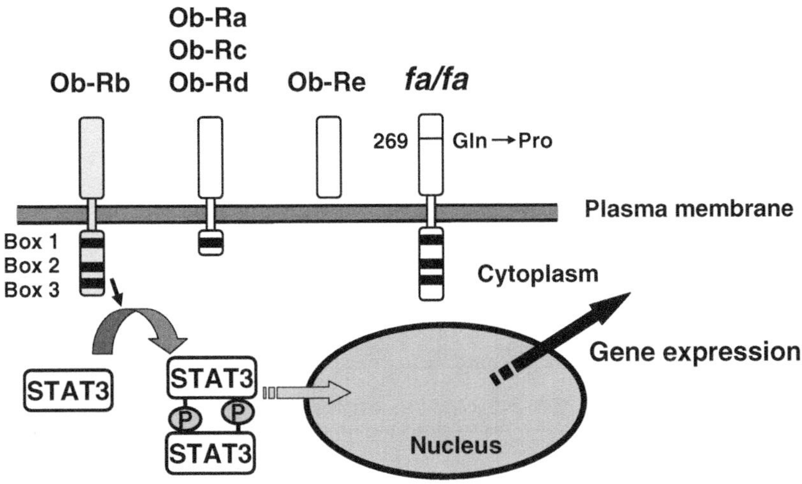

Fig. 1. Isoforms of leptin receptors (Ob-R). *Ob-Ra*, short-form Ob-R; *Ob-Rb*, long-form Ob-R.

leptin augments the inflammation and fibrogenesis in the liver caused by hepatotoxic xenobiotics [4]. These findings lead to the hypothesis that leptin plays a pivotal role in profibrogenic responses in the liver.

Leptin receptors (Ob-R) were originally shown in hypothalamic neurons, through which leptin regulates food intake and body weight [5]. In fact, homozygous mutations of the leptin receptor gene have been identified in rodents (i.e., db/db mice and Zucker rats), which are also associated with obesity [6, 7]. There are several isoforms of Ob-R, which are splice variants with the same extracellular domain. The most ubiquitous form of Ob-R is a short-form receptor (Ob-Ra); however, the function of this receptor isoform remains unclear. In contrast, a long-form leptin receptor (Ob-Rb), which contains a longer intracellular domain, is known to activate the Janus kinase (JAK)-STAT-3 pathway, leading to the transcriptional regulation of target genes (Fig. 1). In the present study, we investigated the expression and functions of Ob-R in hepatic sinusoidal cells in order to elucidate the mechanisms underlying the profibrogenic action of leptin in the liver.

Poor Hepatic Fibrogenesis in Leptin- and Ob-R-Deficient Animals

In a previous study, we [4], demonstrated that administration of recombinant leptin augmented profibrogenic responses in the liver caused by xenobiotics (i.e., carbon tetrachloride and thioacetamide [TAA]) in mice. These observations led us to investigate whether endogenous leptin promoted hepatic fibrogenesis. To answer this question, we utilized ob/ob mice, which lack leptin due to naturally occurring disruption of the leptin gene. Interestingly, ob/ob mice demonstrate extremely poor profibrogenic responses to xenobiotic treatment [8], suggesting that leptin is one of the key regulators of hepatic fibrogenesis.

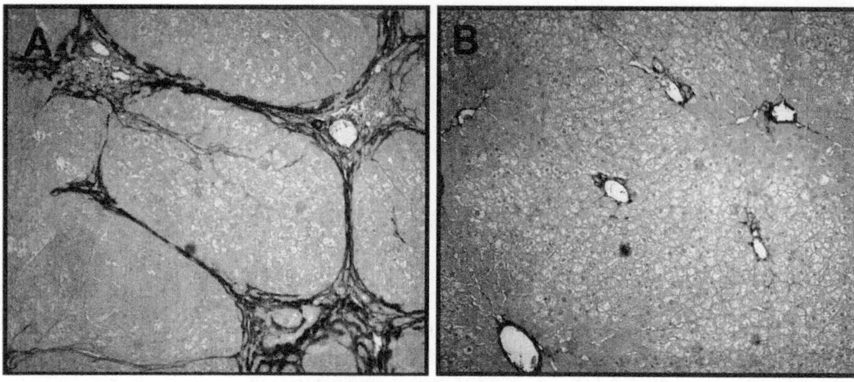

Fig. 2A,B. Thioacetamide (TAA)-induced hepatic fibrosis in Zucker (fa/fa) rats. Male Zucker (fa/fa) rats and their lean littermates (+/?) were given repeated intraperitoneal injections of TAA, (200 mg/kg body weight [BW], three times/week) for 8 weeks, and liver histology was assessed by picro-sirius red staining. **A** Control rats (+/?) treated with TAA. **B** Zucker (fa/fa) rats given TAA. ×40.

Next, we evaluated the role of Ob-R in hepatic fibrogenesis, using Zucker (fa/fa) rats, which lack functional Ob-R due to a missense mutation in the common, extracellular domain [9]. Zucker rats presented extremely poor profibrogenic responses in the liver caused by chronic TAA treatment as compared to their lean littermates (Fig. 2), indicating that Ob-R is involved in the profibrogenic response in the liver. Overt expression of α smooth muscle actin (SMA) in the liver was observed in lean littermates given TAA, whereas αSMA staining was almost negative in Zucker rats even when they were treated with the equivalent amount of TAA. In clear contrast, HSCs isolated from Zucker rats transactivated in vitro were almost the same as the cells isolated from their lean littermates, in terms of the induction of αSMA and steady-state mRNA levels of α1(I)procollagen. This discrepancy in HSC transactivation in vivo and in vitro led us to investigate the expression of Ob-R isoforms in sinusoidal cells.

Sinusoidal Endothelial Cells and Kupffer Cells Express a Functional Ob-R

To determine whether sinusoidal cells express Ob-R isoforms, mRNA for Ob-Ra and Ob-Rb were detected by reverse transcription-polymerase chain reaction (RT-PCR). As expected, Ob-Ra mRNA was detected ubiquitously in HSCs and sinusoidal endothelial cells (SECs). In contrast, Ob-Rb was detected clearly only in SECs and Kupffer cells, but not in 7-day cultured HSCs. Next, to confirm the expression of functional receptors, phosphorylation of STAT-3 was measured by Western blotting. Tyrosine phosphorylation of STAT-3 was clearly detected in SECs when they were treated with leptin (100 nM) for 1 h. In sharp contrast, STAT-3 phosphorylation was barely detectable in rat HSCs even they were incubated with the same dose of leptin. These findings indicated that primary cultured rat SECs express both Ob-Ra and functional

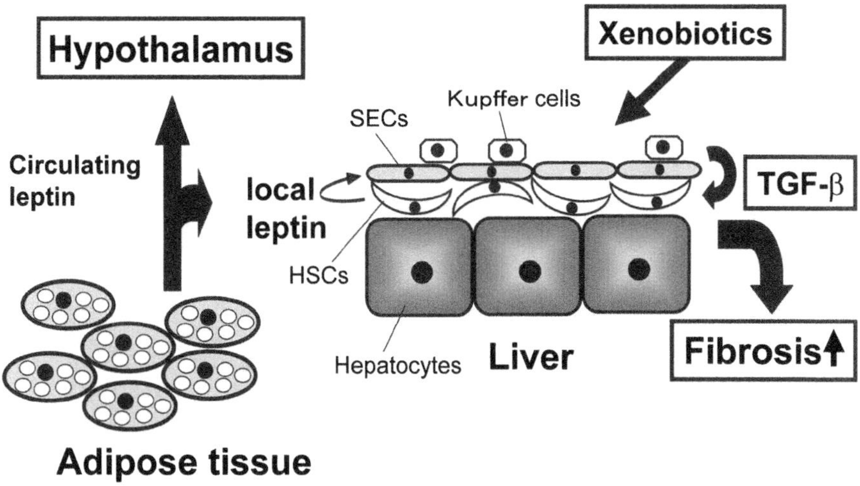

Fig. 3. Leptin is involved in hepatic fibrogenesis: working hypothesis. *SECs*, sinusoidal endothelial cells; *HSCs*, hepatic stellate cells; *TGF-β*, transforming growth factor-β.

Ob-Rb constitutively. Kupffer cells are also positive for the constitutive expression of Ob-Rb. Isolated HSCs, however, appear to express only Ob-Ra, but not Ob-Rb.

Next, we examined whether leptin activated the activator protein (AP)-1 DNA binding in isolated Kupffer cells. The addition of leptin to the medium for 1h increased AP-1 DNA binding activity in a dose-dependent manner. Further, the effect of leptin on steady-state levels of mRNA for transforming growth factor (TGF)-β1 mRNA in Kupffer cells was measured by ribonuclease protection assay. TGF-β1 mRNA levels increased nearly twofold over controls 3–6h after leptin treatment (100nM). Similar, increases in AP-1 DNA binding activity and steady-state mRNA levels of TGF-β1 were observed in LSE cells, a human sinusoidal endothelial cell-derived cell line [9]. In contrast, leptin did not increase steady-state mRNA levels of TGF-β1 in isolated HSCs [8]. Collectively, these observations indicate that leptin most likely upregulates the transcriptional activities of the TGF-β1 gene in Kupffer cells and SECs through the activation of AP-1. It is hypothesized that Ob-Rb-mediated signaling, which is predominant in Kupffer cells and SECs, upregulates the production/activation of TGF-β, thereby facilitating tissue repair and profibrogenic responses in the sinusoidal microenvironment (Fig. 3).

Leptin Facilitates the Proliferation of Hepatic Stellate Cells

As stated above, we have observed that HSCs isolated from Ob-R-deficient Zucker (fa/fa) rats undergo an almost normal transactivation process in vitro [9], suggesting that Ob-R in HSCs is not essential for their activation. On the other hand, emerging lines of evidence suggest the possibility that leptin affects collagen synthesis in isolated HSCs [10]. In line with these observations, we investigated the effect of leptin on the proliferation of HSCs in vitro. The proliferation of 3-day cultured rat HSCs was

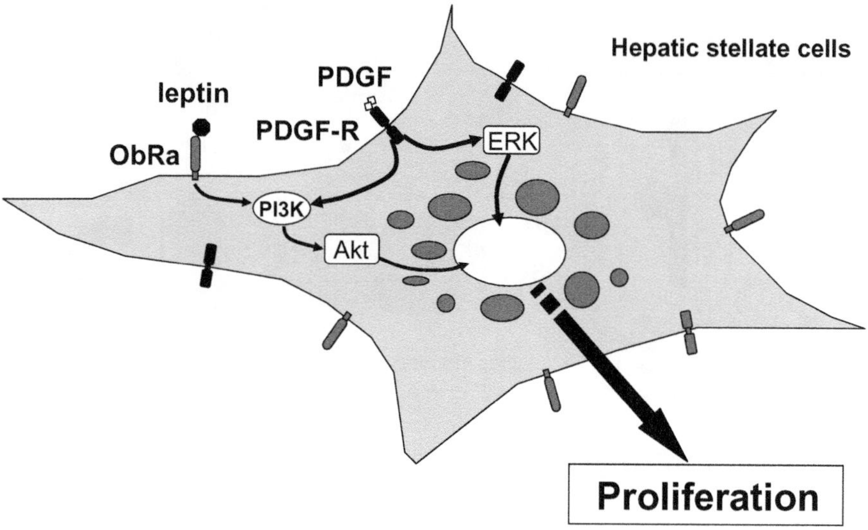

Fig. 4. Leptin enhances platelet-derived growth factor (*PDGF*)-dependent proliferative responses in hepatic stellate cells.

assessed by the incorporation of 5-bromo-2′-deoxyuridine (BrdU) into the nuclei. The percentages of BrdU-positive cells were increased in the presence of platelet-derived growth factor (PDGF)-BB (5 ng/ml) for 8 h, as expected. Co-incubation with leptin (10–100 nM) potentiated this PDGF-dependent increase in BrdU-positive cells in a dose-dependent manner. Messenger RNA for PDGF receptor α and β subunits was increased almost two- to threefold by incubation with leptin for 6 h. Further, preincubation with leptin for 6 h enhanced PDGF-induced increases in phospho-p44/42 mitogen activated protein (MAP) kinase and phospho-Akt levels in a dose-dependent manner. In the same condition, however, leptin per se did not increase phospho-STAT 3 and phospho-p44/42 MAP kinase levels. Instead, leptin increased phospho-Akt levels in HSCs within 30 min, suggesting that the phosphatidylinositol 3 kinase (PI3K)/Akt pathway is involved in the mechanism by which leptin accelerates the proliferation of HSCs (Fig. 4). Taken together, these findings clearly indicate that leptin potentiates the PDGF-dependent proliferative responses of HSCs in vitro.

Conclusion

Leptin and its functional receptors play a crucial role in hepatic fibrogenesis, most likely through the upregulation of TGF-β expression in the liver. Further, leptin augments PDGF-dependent proliferative responses in HSCs, most likely through actions involving the PI3K/Akt pathway. On the other hand, it is likely that leptin ameliorates hepatic steatosis and inflammatory responses. Taken together, these findings suggest that leptin can be characterized as a tissue-repairing cytokine (Fig. 5). In conclusion, it is postulated that leptin, produced systemically from adipose tissue and locally from

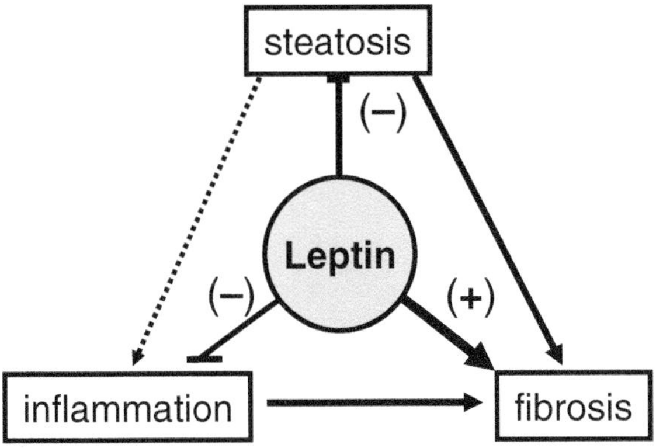

Fig. 5. Role of leptin in progression of steatohepatitis.

HSCs, contributes to the progression of hepatic fibrosis in a variety of obesity-related chronic liver diseases, including NASH.

References

1. Zhang Y, Proenca R, Maffei M, Barone M, Leopold L, Friedman JM (1994) Positional cloning of the mouse obese gene and its human homologue. Nature 372: 425–432
2. McCullough AJ, Bugianesi E, Marchesini G, Kalhan SC (1998) Gender dependent alterations in serum leptin in alcoholic cirrhosis. Gastroenterology 115: 947–953
3. Potter JJ, Womack L, Mezey E, Anania FA (1998) Transdifferentiation of rat hepatic stellate cells results in leptin expression. Biochem Biophys Res Commun 244: 178–182
4. Ikejima K, Honda H, Yoshikawa M, Hirose M, Kitamura T, Takei Y, Sato N (2001) Leptin augments inflammatory and profibrogenic responses in the murine liver induced by hepatotoxic chemicals. Hepatology 34: 288–297
5. Tartaglia LA, Dembski M, Weng X, Deng N, Culpepper J, Devos R, Richards GJ, Campfield LA, Clark FT, Deeds J, Muir C, Sanker S, Moriarty A, Moore KJ, Smutko JS, Mays GG, Woolf EA, Monroe CA, Tepper RI (1995) Identification and expression cloning of a leptin receptor Ob-R. Cell 83: 1263–1271
6. Lee GH, Proenca R, Montez JM, Carroll KM, Darvishzadeh HG, Lee JI, Friedman JM (1996) Abnormal splicing of the leptin receptor in diabetic mice. Nature 379: 632–635
7. Takaya K, Ogawa Y, Isse N, Okazaki T, Satoh N, Masuzaki H, Mori K, Tamura N, Hosoda K, Nakao K (1996) Molecular cloning of rat leptin receptor isoform complementary DNAs—identification of a missense mutation in Zucker fatty (fa/fa) rats. Biochem. Biophys. Res. Commun. 225: 75–83
8. Honda H, Ikejima K, Hirose M, Yoshikawa M, Lang T, Enomoto N, Kitamura T, Takei Y, Sato N (2002) Leptin is required for fibrogenic responses induced by thioacetamide in the murine liver. Hepatology 36: 12–21
9. Ikejima K, Takei Y, Honda H, Hirose M, Yoshikawa M, Zhang YJ, Lang T, Fukuda T, Yamashina S, Kitamura T, Sato N (2002) Leptin receptor-mediated signaling regulates hepatic fibrogenesis and remodeling of extracellular matrix in the rat. Gastroenterology 122: 1399–1410
10. Saxena NK, Ikeda K, Rockey DC, Friedman SL, Anania FA (2002) Leptin in hepatic fibrosis: evidence for increased collagen production in stellate cells and lean littermates of ob/ob mice. Hepatology 35: 762–771

Zone 3 Predominance of Histopathological Features in Nonalcoholic Steatohepatitis

Hideaki Enzan, Makoto Toi, Yoshihiro Hayashi, Tadashi Hamauzu, Naoto Kuroda, and Makoto Hiroi

Summary. Nonalcoholic steatohepatitis (NASH) has a wide spectrum of histopathological features in terms of the necroinflammatory grading and the staging of fibrosis. Among these features, steatosis, necroinflammatory changes in the acinus (lobular hepatitis), and fibrosis show a definite zonal heterogeneity in liver acini; namely, a zone-3 predominance. Macrovesicular liver-cell steatosis is usually seen in zone 3. Ballooning degeneration and Mallory's hyaline are predominantly observed in liver cells in acinar zone 3, and the activation of Kupffer's cells and hepatic stellate cells (HSCs) is also present in zone 3. The basic and initial fibrosis that characterizes NASH also occurs in zone 3. This zone-3 predominance from the initial features through to the subsequent fibrosis in NASH suggests that injurious process(es) preferentially hit liver cells in zone 3. Based on the excessive deposition of neutral fat, cytochrome P450 (CYP) 2E1 may be induced, associated with the influence of other factors. The activated enzyme may generate free radicals, initiating lipid peroxidation. The aldehyde metabolites of lipid peroxidation may cause lobular hepatitis. Following the liver cell necrosis that occurs due to the inflammation, zone-3 fibrosis initially develops, associated with the activation of HSCs in that location. These sequential events that occur predominantly in zone 3 may, in part, reflect the complicated pathogensis of NASH.

Key words. NASH, Histopathology, Liver acinus, Hepatic stellate cell, Zone 3 fibrosis

Introduction

Nonalcoholic steatohepatitis (NASH), a liver disease defined by both clinical (nonalcoholic) and histopathological (steatohepatitis) characteristics [1–3], is a common form of chronic fibrotic disease. Needle-biopsied liver tissues obtained from patients with NASH show varied appearances from patient to patient in the extent of histopathological changes and their zonal distribution in liver acini. The main histopathological findings are roughly classified into four categories; liver cell steatosis-associated findings, necroinflammatory changes in acini (lobular hepatitis) and in portal tracts (portal hepatitis), and fibrosis of various degrees. The first category includes macrovesicular liver-cell steatosis, fatty cysts, and glycogenated nuclei

Department of Pathology, Program of Bioregulation and Genetics, Kochi Medical School, Kochi University, Kohasu, Oko-cho, Nankoku, Kochi 783-8505, Japan of liver cells. The features of lobular hepatitis consist of liver-cell degeneration, except for fatty changes and liver-cell necrosis. Liver cells with ballooning degeneration, Mallory's hyaline, and siderosis appear. Single-cell death and focal necrosis of liver cells are seen in a scattered pattern. Ultrastructurally, megamitochondria with paracrystalline inclusions are occasionally observed in liver cells. Activation of Kupffer cells and hepatic stellate cells (HSCs) also occurs. Chronic and acute inflammatory cells infiltrate the liver acini. In addition to these features of lobular hepatitis, features of portal hepatitis may also be present, although the changes are less marked than those in lobular hepatitis. The continued presence of liver cell necrosis and inflammation leads to fibrosis, predominantly intraacinar in location, and this gradually increases in severity and distribution, until cryptogenic liver cirrhosis occurs [4–6].

The aim of the present chapter is to demonstrate the zonal heterogeneity of various histopathological finding in liver acini; namely, a zone-3 predominance, and to show the changes of HSCs, with reference to liver fibrosis, in patients with NASH.

Zonal Heterogeneity of Histopathological Findings in Liver Acini in NASH

Table 1 summarizes the main histopathological findings in NASH and the zone predominantly involved in liver acini. According to Brunt et al. [2] and Brunt [3], steatosis (predominantly macrovesicular), mild mixed lobular inflammation (which includes scattered polymorphonuclear leukocytes, as well as mononuclear cells), and hepatocellular ballooning are necessarily present as components of NASH. Perisinusoidal fibrosis, glycogenated nuclei of liver cells, lipogranulomas, acidophil bodies, d-PAS-positive Kupffer's cells, and fatty cysts are usually present, but are not necessary for diagnosis. Mallory's hyaline and iron deposition, as well as megamitochondria in liver cells, may be present, but these also are not necessary for diagnosis.

It is generally accepted that NASH has a wide spectrum of histopathological features in terms of necroinflammatory grading and staging of the fibrosis [2, 3], although diffuse involvement of the liver is common. In early-stage and mild cases of NASH, significant steatosis of liver cells, with mild lobular inflammation, but without any evidence of fibrosis, may be present [2]. Active and severe cases of NASH may show almost all the findings listed in Table 1, and in such cases, it is not difficult to make a histopathological diagnosis of NASH or steatohepatitis. With progression of the disease, the livers in patients with NASH show increased fibrosis stage [2, 3], associated with the architectural distortion of the acinus, and the condition ultimately develops to cryptogenic cirrhosis [4–6].

In NASH, most of the histopathological features in liver acini, show a relatively clear zonal heterogeneity in intensity, possibly reflected the underlying pathogenesis. With the progression of NASH, the histopathological features extend into adjacent zones and occasionally to all acinar zones, resulting in the disappearance of the zonal heterogeneity of the features. The macrovesicular steatosis that characterizes NASH is predominantly present in acinar zone-3 liver cells, with initial relative sparing of zone 1 [3]. In some cases the steatosis extends beyond zone 3 into zones 2 and 1. On the other hand, the hepatic steatosis may almost disappear after the development of cirrhosis [4–6]. Glycogenated nuclei are usually seen in nonsteatotic liver cells in zone 1

Table 1. The main histopathological lesions and the acinar zone predominantly involved in NASH

Lesions	Acinar zone predominantly involved
1. Steatosis—associated lesions	
Liver cell steatosis (predominantly macrovesicular)	In zone 3 [2, 3]
Fatty cysts	
Glycogenated nuclei of liver cells	Preferentially in zone 1 [2, 3]
2. Lobular hepatitis—associated lesions	
Liver cell degeneration, except for fatty changes and necrosis	
Ballooning degeneration	In zone 3 [3]
Mallory's hyaline	In zone 3 [3]
Single-cell death (acidophil bodies)	
Focal necrosis	
Megamitochondria with paracrystalline inclusions	
Iron deposition in liver cells	Zone 1 [3]
Induction of cytochrome *P*450 2E1 in liver cells	Zone 3 [7]
Lipid peroxidation product (HNE) in liver cells	Zone 3 [12]
Lipogranuloma (fat granuloma)	
Kupffer cell activation	Zone 3 [13]
Ceroid macrophages	
Activation of hepatic stellate cells	Zone 3 [16, 17]
Chronic and acute inflammatory cell infiltrates	
Neutrophils	Frequently seen around degenerated liver cells with Mallory's hyaline [2, 3]
3. Portal hepatitis—associated lesions	
4. Fibrosis	
Perivenular	
Pericellular and/or perisinusoidal	Zone 3 [2, 3]

NASH, nonalcoholic steatohepatitis; HNE, 4-Hydroxy-2′-nonenal

[2, 3] and are never seen in steatotic liver cells in zone 3. According to Brunt [3], ballooning degeneration is most apparent near steatotic liver cells, typically in zone 3. Mallory's hyaline, when present, is located in the ballooned hepatocytes in zone 3. Granular iron deposition is reported in liver cells in zone 1, although NASH cases in Japan usually show no or mild iron deposition. Immunohistochemistry of formalin-fixed, paraffin-embedded needle liver biopsy sections demonstrates the distribution of cytochrome P450 (CYP) 2E1 (the principal microsomal catalyst of lipid peroxidation) [7, 8], or the distribution of microsomal lipoxygenase [9]. In normal human livers, the enzyme distribution is confined to a thin layer, two to three cells thick, around the terminal hepatic venules [7]. In NASH, immunostaining for CYP 2E1 shows an intense staining pattern in zone 3 extending into zone 2, corresponding to the acinar distribution of steatosis [7] (Fig. 1). The increased CYP 2E1 activity may contribute to the development and progression of necroinflammatory changes (lobular hepatitis) in NASH, through the increased production of free radicals, initiating significant lipid peroxidation [10]. The highly reactive aldehyde products of lipid peroxidation, 4-hydroxy-2′-nonenal (HNE) and malondialdehyde (MDA), are capable

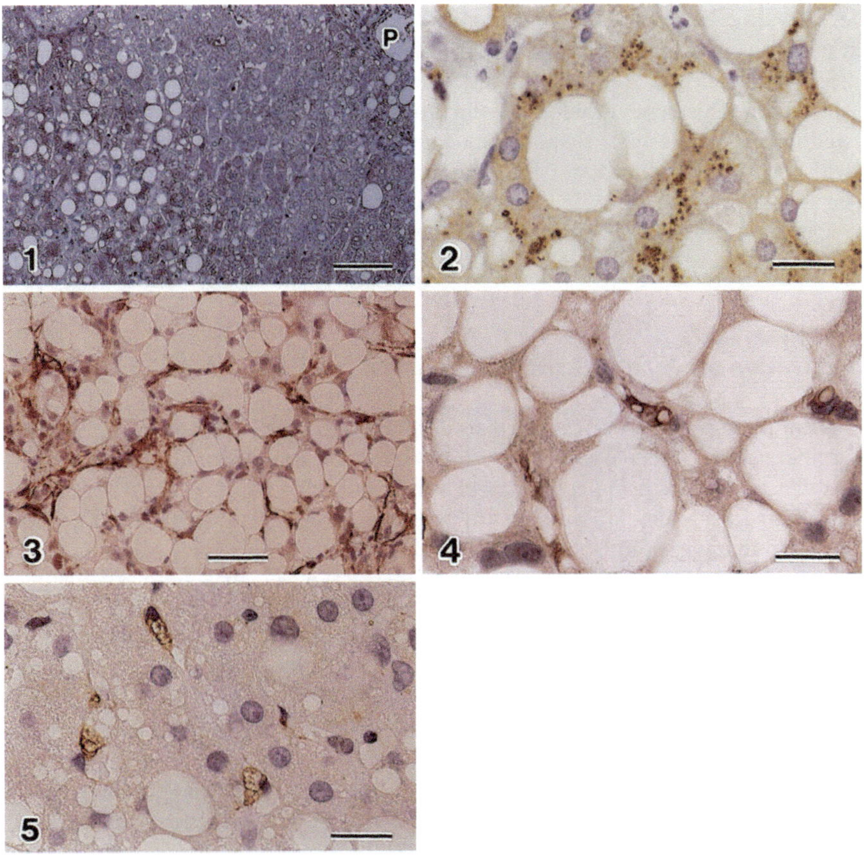

Fig. 1. Liver section from a patient with nonalcoholic steatohepatitis (NASH). Immunostaining for cytochrome P450 (CYP) 2E1. The immunostaining for CYP 2E1 is intense in steatotic liver cells in zone 3 (*left lower half of Fig.*), while nonsteatotic liver cells in zone 1 (*right upper half*) are negative for CYP 2E1. *P*, portal tract. *Scale bar*, 100 μm.

Fig. 2. Liver section from a patient with NASH. Immunostaining for 4-hydroxy-2′-nonenal (HNE). HNE is mainly detected in steatotic liver cells in zone 3. *Scale bar*, 20 μm.

Fig. 3. Liver section from a patient with NASH. Immunostaining for α-smooth muscle actin (SMA). In the area of zone-3 fibrosis, α-SMA-positive hepatic stellate cells (HSCs) are increased in number and become spindle-shaped, showing a myofibroblast-like transformation. *Scale bar*, 50 μm.

Fig. 4. Liver section from a patient with NASH. Immunostaining for leptin. HSCs adjacent to steatotic liver cells in zone 3 are positive for leptin, although they contain a few fat droplets. *Scale bar*, 20 μm.

Fig. 5. Liver section from a patient with NASH. Immunostaining for α-smooth muscle actin (α-SMA). Adjacent to steatotic liver cells, α-SMA-positive hepatic stellate cells are seen, but they are enlarged and contain some small fat droplets. *Scale bar*, 20 μm.

of activating HSCs [10, 11], cross-linking cytokeratins to form Mallory's hyaline, and stimulating neutrophil chemotaxis. MDA may also contribute to the inflammation by activating nuclear factor (NF)-κB [10]. In cases of NASH, HNE, one of the most reliable immunohistochemical markers for peroxidation, is widely detected, and is localized in the cytoplasm of steatotic hepatocytes (Fig. 2), as well as in sinusoidal cells, with a predominance in zone 3 [12], although no immunostaining for HNE is observed in normal human livers. In cases of steatohepatitis, Kupffer's cells in perivenular regions are prominently enlarged and aggregated, while those in zones 2 and 1 are neither enlarged nor aggregated; the appearance of individual Kupffer's cells in these zones is identical to that in normal livers [13].

Activation of Hepatic Stellate Cells and Zone 3 Fibrosis

In liver fibrosis, after liver-cell necrosis occurs, adjacent HSCs are promptly activated, proliferate, and undergo phenotypic transformation from vitamin A-storing cells (a feature of HSCs in the quiescent stage) into myofibroblast-like cells that express positive immunostaining for α-smooth muscle actin (α-SMA)[14] (Fig. 3). It is generally accepted that the α-SMA-positive activated HSCs become the principal cells involved in producing almost all components of the extracellular matrix and participating in liver fibrosis, regardless of the etiology. Activated HSCs can also express leptin [15] (Fig. 4). In cases of NASH, the number of activated HSCs is increased in zone 3 [16, 17]. A clear correlation between the degree of HSC activation and lobular and portal inflammation is reported [17]. In most cases, the degree of HSC activation parallels the degree of hepatic fibrosis [16]. However, α-SMA-positive HSCs simultaneously showing features of the quiescent and the activated stages of the cells are occasionally seen in zone 3 (Fig. 5). The pathological significance of such HSCs, having both activated and quiescent features (α-SMA-positive HSCs with some small intracyto-

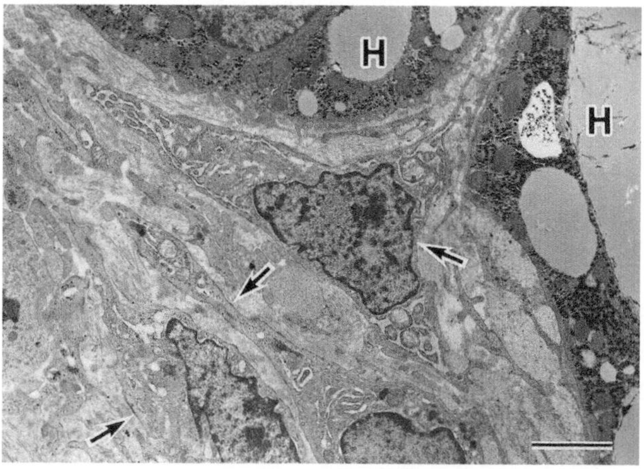

Fig. 6. Liver section from a patient with NASH. Activated HSCs, showing myofibroblast-like transformation in zone-3 fibrosis. In the cytoplasm, well-developed rough-surfaced endoplasmic reticulum and Golgi complex are present. Along the cell membrane, dense bodies are frequently seen. *Arrows* indicate activated HSCs. *H*, steatotic liver cell. *Scale bar*, 3 μm.

plasmic fat droplets containing vitamin A) is not yet clear. Fig. 6 shows the ultrastructure of activated HSCs. According to the fibrosis staging for NASH proposed by Brunt et al. [2] and Brunt [3], in stage 0, no fibrosis is present in livers. Stage 1 patients show zone-3 perisinusoidal/pericellular fibrosis, which is either focal or extensive (Fig. 7a, c, d). In stage 2, there is periportal fibrosis of varying degrees, and in stage 3 there is central-central (C-C), and portal-central (P-C) bridging fibrosis (Fig. 7b). The

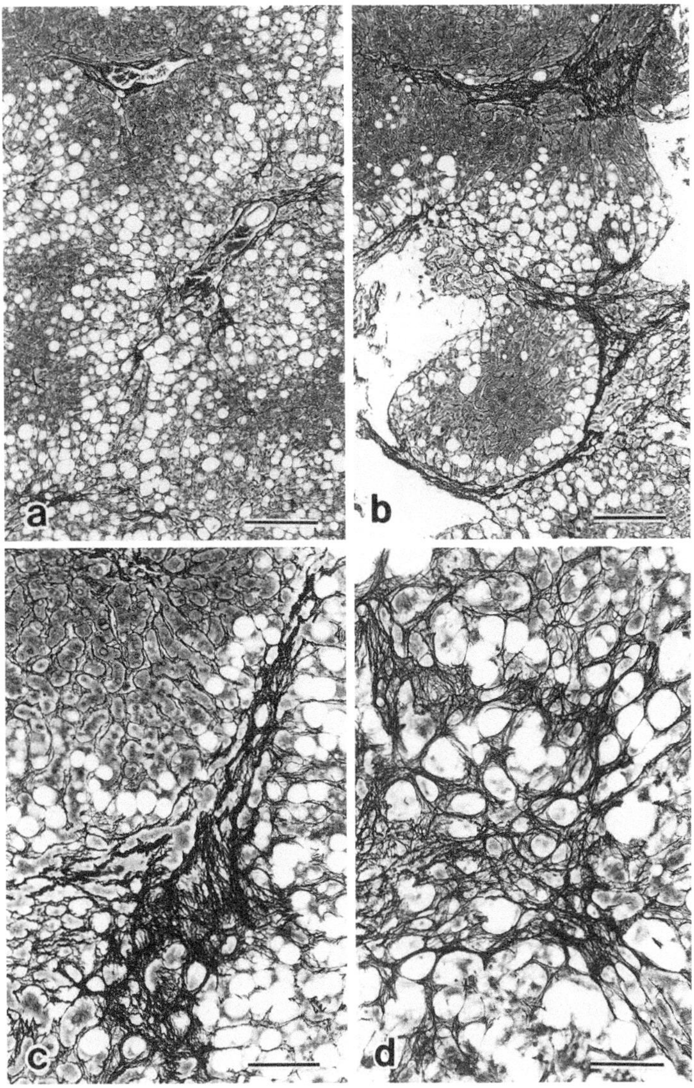

Fig. 7a–d. Liver sections from patients with NASH; silver impregnation, showing lower magnification (**a** and **b**) and higher magnification (**c** and **d**) of fibrotic lesions. **a** Shows stage 1, with zone-3 fibrosis; **b** shows stage 3, with central-central (C-C) bridging fibrosis as well as portal fibrosis. **c** and **d** Show zone-3 fibrosis of various degrees and patterns. **a** and **b**, *Scale bars*, 200 μm; **c** and **d**, *scale bars*, 100 μm.

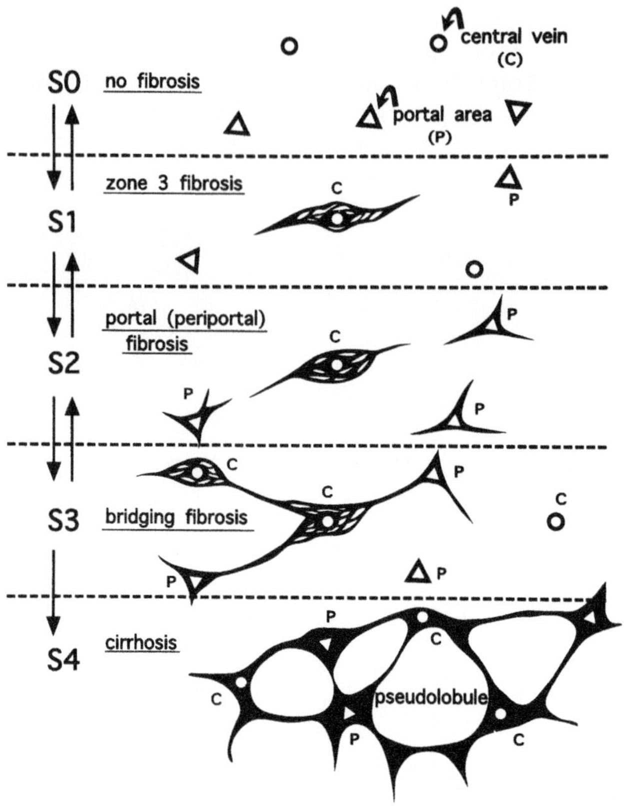

Fig. 8. Schematic presentation of fibrosis staging in NASH. Zone-3 fibrosis is the initial and basic pattern of fibrosis in NASH, and it contrasts markedly with the periportal and portal-based fibrosis seen in chronic viral hepatitis. *S*, stage.

causes of the periportal fibrosis seen in various degrees in stage 2 remain unclear. Stage 4 is the stage of cirrhosis (Fig. 8).

Conclusions

The livers of patients with NASH show a wide spectrum of histopathological features. Most of the features show definite zonal heterogeneity; namely, predominance in zone 3, compared with findings in zones 1 and 2. This suggests that the initial and major injurious process(es) in NASH may hit liver cells in zone 3, resulting in significant liver-cell steatosis. Based on the liver-cell steatosis, CYP 2E1 may be induced through the disturbance of lipid metabolism. The activated enzyme may generate free radicals, initiating lipid peroxidation. The cytotoxic lipid peroxidation byproducts may then cause inflammation in that location. After the liver-cell necrosis that occurs due to the inflammation, the zone-3 fibrosis that characterizes NASH occurs, associated with the activation of HSCs. These sequential events may reflect the multiple factors involved, and the complicated pathogenesis of NASH.

References

1. Ludwig J, Viggiano TR, Mcgill DB, Ott BJ (1980) Nonalcoholic steatohepatitis, Mayo Clinic experiences with a hitherto unnamed disease. Mayo Clin Proc 55: 434–438
2. Brunt EM, Janney CG, Bisceglie AMD, Neuschwandler-Tetri BA, Bacon BR (1999) Nonalcoholic steatohepatitis: a proposal for grading and staging the histological lesions. Am J Gastroenterol 94: 2467–2474
3. Brunt EM (2001) Nonalcoholic steatohepatitis: definition and pathology. Semin Liver Dis 21:3–16
4. Caldwell SH, Oelsner DH, Iezzoni JC, Hespenheide EE, Battle EH, Driscoll CJ (1999) Cryptogenic cirrhosis: clinical characterization and risk factors for underlying disease. Hepatology 29: 664–669
5. Contos MJ, Sanyal AJ (2002) The clinicopathologic spectrum and management of nonalcoholic fatty liver disease. Adv Anat Pathol 9: 37–51
6. Ayata G, Gordon FD, Lewis WD, Pomfret E, Pomposelli JJ, Jenkins RL, Khettry U (2002) Cryptogenic cirrhosis: clinicopathologic findings at and after liver transplantation. Hum Pathol 33: 1098–1104
7. Weltman MD, Farrell GC, Hall P, Ingelman-Sundberg M, Liddle C (1998) Hepatic cytochrome P450 2E1 is increased in patients with nonalcoholic steatohepatitis. Hepatology 27: 128–133
8. Leclercq IA, Farrell GC, Field J, Bell DR, Gonzalez FJ, Robertson GR (2000) CYP2E1 and CYP4A as microsomal catalysts of lipid peroxides in murine nonalcoholic steatohepatitis. J Clin Invest 105: 1067–1075
9. Chitturi S, Farrell GC (2001) Etiopathogenesis of nonalcoholic steatohepatitis. Semin Liver Dis 21: 27–41
10. Day CP (1998) Steatohepatitis: a tale of two 'hits'. Gastroenterology 114: 842–845
11. Parola M, Pinzani M, Casini A, Albano E, Poli G, Gentilini A, Gentilini P, Dianzani MU (1993) Stimulation of lipid peroxidation or 4-hydroxynonenal treatment increases procollagen $\alpha 1$(I) gene expression in human liver fat-storing cells. Biochem Biophys Res Commun 194: 1044–1050
12. Seki S, Kitada T, Yamada T, Sakaguchi H, Nakatani K, Wakasa K (2002) In situ detection of lipid peroxidation and oxidative DNA damage in non-alcoholic fatty liver diseases. J Hepatol 37: 56–62
13. Lefkowitch JH, Haythe JH, Regent N (2002) Kupffer cell aggregation and perivenular distribution in steatohepatitis. Mod Pathol 15: 699–704
14. Enzan H, Himeno H, Iwamura S, Saibara T, Onishi S, Yamamoto Y, Hara H (1994) Immunohistochemical identification of Ito cells and their myofibroblastic transformation in adult human liver. Virchows Arch 424: 249–256
15. Potter JJ, Womack L, Mezey E, Anania FA (1998) Transdifferentiation of rat hepatic stellate cells results in leptin expression. Biochem Biophys Res Commun 244: 178–182
16. Washington K, Wright K, Shyr Y, Hunter EB, Olson S, Raiford DS (2000) Hepatic stellate cell activation in nonalcoholic steatohepatitis and fatty liver. Hum Pathol 31: 822–828
17. Cortez-Pinto H, Baptista A, Camilo ME, de Moura MC (2001) Hepatic stellate cell activation occurs in nonalcoholic steatohepatitis. Hepato-gastroenterology 48: 87–90

Genetic Background of Japanese Patients with Nonalcoholic Steatohepatitis (NASH)

Toshiji Saibara[1], Chikako Namikawa[1], Zhang Shu-Ping[1], Ma Rui-Hong[1], Yasuko Nozaki[1], Yoshihisa Nemoto[1], Masafumi Ono[1], Naoaki Akisawa[1], Shinji Iwasaki[1], Makoto Hiroi[2], Hideaki Enzan[2], and Saburo Onishi[1]

Summary. The pathogenesis of nonalcoholic steatohepatitis (NASH) is not understood well. Therefore, it is necessary to examine genetic influences on NASH pathogenesis. Two functional polymorphisms were studied: the −493 G/T polymorphism in the promoter of microsomal triglyceride transfer protein (MTP) and the 1183 T/C polymorphism in the mitochondrial targeting sequence of manganese superoxide dismutase (MnSOD). The G allele in the MTP promoter leads to decreased MTP transcription, less export of triglyceride from hepatocytes, and greater intracellular triglyceride accumulation. In addition, glucose intolerance with hyperinsulinemia, which may be responsible for down-regulating *MTP* mRNA expression, is frequent among NASH patients, as observed in caucasians. The T allele in the MnSOD mitochondrial targeting sequence leads to less transport of MnSOD to the mitochondria. Blood samples from patients with biopsy-proven NASH and healthy controls were analyzed by the polymerase chain reaction (PCR) and restriction fragment length polymorphism (RFLP). Functional polymorphisms in MTP and MnSOD were revealed to be involved in determining susceptibility to NASH in Japanese.

Key words. Fatty liver, Single-nucleotide polymorphism, Manganese-SOD, Microsomal triglyceride transfer protein, Obesity

Introduction

The term "nonalcoholic steatohepatitis (NASH)" is used to describe a form of liver injury that is indistinguishable from alcoholic hepatitis [1]. The pathological features of NASH reveal hepatic steatosis with hepatocellular injury, focal mixed cell-type inflammation, and fibrosis [2, 3]. In fact, most cases of NASH appear to have a multifactorial etiopathogenesis. Current models propose a "two-hit" hypothesis, whereby lipid first accumulates in hepatocytes, then triggers inflammation by a variety of mechanisms [4]. Accumulated data support this idea. For example, obesity was found in half of a cohort of patients with cryptogenic cirrhosis [5].

[1] Department of Gastroenterology and Hepatology, Kochi Medical School, Kohasu, Oko-cho, Nankoku, Kochi 783-8505, Japan
[2] Department of Pathology, Kochi Medical School, Kohasu, Oko-cho, Nankoku, Kochi 783-8505, Japan

Genetic variation in lipid metabolism may produce differences in the speed and extent of hepatocyte lipid accumulation, the "first hit." One relevant enzyme is the microsomal triglyceride transfer protein (MTP). This protein transfers triglycerides to nascent apolipoprotein B, producing very-low-density lipoprotein (VLDL) and removing lipid from the hepatocyte. Patients with abetalipoproteinemia, an autosomal recessive disease caused by mutations in the MTP coding region, develop marked hepatic steatosis early in life [6]. *MTP* mRNA expression in human hepatocytes is downregulated by insulin (7).

There is considerable evidence for the role of oxidative damage in NASH, one of the "second hits". In a steatotic liver, free fatty acids are diverted to the mitochondria, where they are oxidized by beta-oxidation, and may generate increased amounts of reactive oxygen species (ROS). Lipid peroxidation likely damages plasma and intracellular membranes, leading to apoptosis and necrosis of hepatocytes. Lipid peroxidation end-products (malondialdehyde and 4-hydroxy-2-nonenal [HNE]) may also trigger inflammatory and immune-mediated mechanisms of hepatocyte injury [8]. Animal models of nonalcoholic fatty liver disease and biopsy specimens of patients with alcoholic liver disease have shown that the degree of lipid peroxidation in the liver correlates with the extent of steatosis.

One enzyme that is important in detoxifying mitochondrial ROS is manganese superoxide dismutase (MnSOD). This enzyme is synthesized in the cytosol and modified post-transcriptionally for transport to the mitochondria [9]. A limited number of polymorphisms have been described for MnSOD, including a T/C polymorphism in the mitochondrial targeting sequence. This polymorphism leads to a valine-to-alanine amino- acid change in the mitochondrial targeting sequence. In turn, this amino-acid substitution may alter the helical structure of the mitochondrial targeting sequence, enhancing the transport of MnSOD into the mitochondrial matrix [10].

Here, we review the importance of hyperinsulinemia and functional polymorphisms of MTP and MnSOD in determining an individual's susceptibility to NASH (Fig. 1).

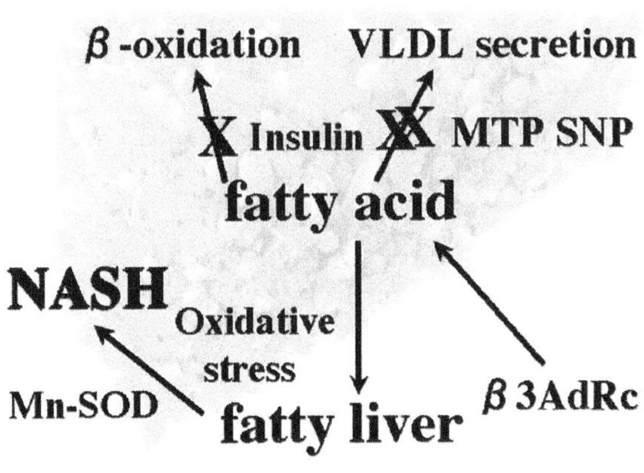

Fig. 1. Fatty acid metabolism pathway in the liver, and the development of hepatic steatosis. *VLDL*, very low density lipoprotein; *MTP*, microsomal triglyceride transfer protein; *SNP*, single-nucleotide polymorphism; *NASH*, nonalcoholic steatohepatitis; *SOD*, superoxide dismutase.

Hyperinsulinemia

NASH is often linked with disorders that are clearly associated with insulin resistance, obesity, hypertriglyceridemia, and type 2 diabetes mellitus. Fasting plasma insulin level is high in two-thirds of NASH patients (Fig. 2). The majority of NASH patients have glucose intolerance when challenged with 75g oral glucose (Fig. 3). This is a frequent observation in western countries; however, glucose intolerance with hyperinsulinemia is an infrequent observation among Japanese, because the majority of glucose intolerance observed in Japanese is associated with impaired insulin secretion. This unusual frequency of hyperinsulinemia in NASH patients reveals the importance of hyperinsulinemia in the development of NASH. It is important to remember that hyperinsulinemia results in downregulated hepatic fatty-acid beta-oxidation and mRNA expression of MTP [7].

Functional–493 G/T Polymorphism in the Promoter of Microsomal Triglyceride Transfer Protein (MTP)

Recently, hepatic steatosis in patients with chronic hepatitis C has attracted much attention. Hepatitis C virus core protein was proved to inhibit MTP activity and VLDL secretion [11]. The G allele has been previously shown to produce less *MTP* gene transcription than the T allele. Less MTP activity would lead to lower excretion of triglyceride as VLDL, and greater accumulation of lipid in the hepatocytes [12]. Thus, the G allele in the MTP promoter would render a patient more susceptible to steatosis,

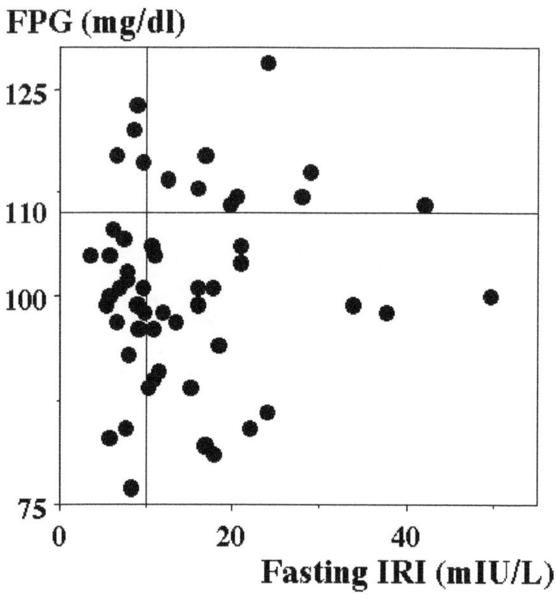

Fig. 2. Levels of fasting plasma glucose (*FPG*) and fasting plasma insulin in NASH patients. *IRI*, immunoreactive insulin.

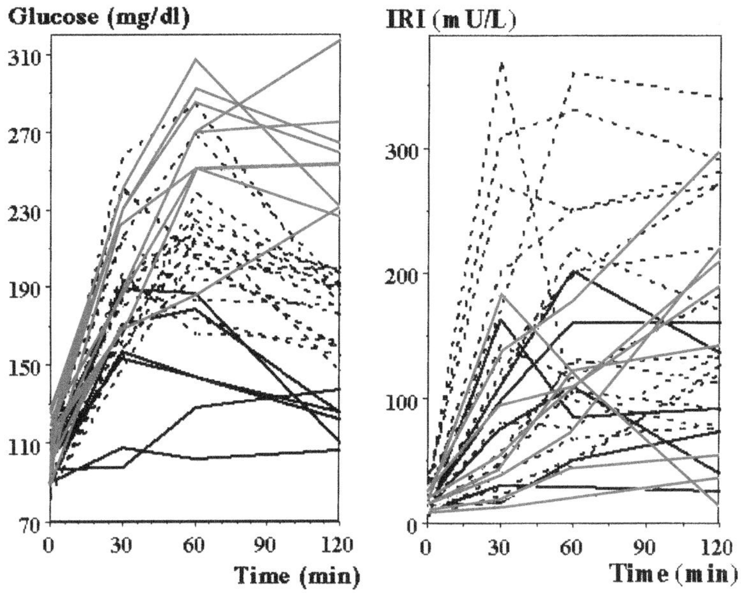

Fig. 3. 75-g Oral glucose tolerance test in NASH patients.

the "first hit" in the "two-hit" hypothesis of NASH pathogenesis. The G/G genotype is observed in 60% of Japanese [13]. The increased susceptibility to steatosis is apparent in a wide population of NASH patients in Japan. The stage of fibrosis, assessed by Brunt's criteria, was significantly higher in NASH patients with the G/G genotype than in patients with the G/T genotype. However, there were no significant differences in terms of age, body mass index (BMI) or levels of alanine aminotransferase (ALT), fasting triglyceride, and total cholesterol between the G/G-genotype and the G/T-genotype groups.

Functional 1183 T/C Polymorphism in the Targeting Sequence of Manganese Superoxide Dismutase (MnSOD)

Excessive oxidative stress has been suggested as the "second hit", by a pathophysiologic molecule, in the development of NASH [14]. MnSOD, a potent scavenger, of oxygen free radicals, localized to mitochondria, has a key role in preventing oxidative stress to hepatocytes. Less effective targeting of MnSOD to mitochondria may affect a patient's susceptibility to NASH, by decreasing the capacity to detoxify superoxide anions produced in mitochondria and increasing the susceptibility to excessive oxidative stress in hepatocytes [15]. In fact, as the T allele results in less effective targeting of MnSOD [16], higher oxidative stress may result in a higher prevalence of NASH. The T/T genotype frequency in NASH patients was found to be significantly higher than that in controls [13]. Unfortunately, the C allele was shown to have a lower prevalence in Japanese than in Chinese and European populations. This may render Japanese people more susceptible to oxidative stress in hepatocytes than other populations.

Conclusions

Severe insulin resistance with hyperinsulinemia is a characteristic clinical feature in Japanese NASH patients, as well as in NASH patients from other ethnic groups, although the majority of Japanese NASH patients have impaired insulin secretion. However, the frequency of Japanese NASH patients with both the G/G genotype of MTP and the T/T genotype of MnSOD was significantly higher than that in healthy volunteers. This may render Japanese more susceptible to oxidative stress in hepatocytes than other populations in the world.

References

1. Ludwig J, Viggiano TR, McGill DB (1980) Nonalcoholic steatohepatitis: Mayo Clinic experiences with a hitherto unnamed disease. Mayo Clin Proc 55: 434–438
2. Brunt EM, Janney CG, Di Bisceglie AM (1999) Nonalcoholic steatohepatitis: a proposal for grading and staging the histological lesions. Am J Gastroenterol 94: 2467–2474
3. Brunt EM (2001) Nonalcoholic steatohepatitis: definition and pathology. Semin Liver Dis 21: 3–16
4. Day CP, James OFW (1998) Steatohepatitis: a tale of two 'hits'? Gastroenterology 114: 842–844
5. Caldwell SH, Oelsner DH, Iezzoni JC (1999) Cryptogenic cirrhosis: clinical characterization and risk factor for underlying disease. Hepatology 29: 664–669
6. Wetterau JR, Lin MC, Jamil H (1997) Microsomal triglyceride transfer protein. Biochim Biophys Acta 1345: 136–150
7. Au WS, Kung HF, Lin MC (2003) Regulation of microsomal triglyceride transfer protein gene by insulin in HepG2 cells. Roles of MAPK/erk and MAPK/p38. Diabetes 52: 1073–1080
8. Day CP, Saksena S (2002) Non-alcoholic steatohepatitis: definitions and pathogenesis. J Gastroenterol Hepatol 17: S377–S384
9. Wispe JR, Clark JC, Burhans MS (1989) Synthesis and processing of the precursor for human mangano-superoxide dismutase. Biochim Biophys Acta 994: 30–34
10. Stewart SF, Leathart JB, Chen Y (2002) Valine-alanine manganese superoxide dismutase polymorphism is not associated with alcohol-induced oxidative stress or liver fibrosis. Hepatology 36: 1355–1360
11. Perlemuter G, Sabile A, Letteron P (2002) Hepatitis C virus core protein inhibits microsomal triglyceride transfer protein activity and very low density lipoprotein secretion: a model of viral-related steatosis. FASEB J 16: 185–194.
12. Bernard S, Touzet S, Personne I (2000) Association between microsomal triglyceride transfer protein gene polymorphism and the biological features of liver steatosis in patients with type II diabetes. Diabetologia 43: 995–999
13. Namikawa C, Zhang S-P, Vyselaar JR, et al. (2004) Polymorphisms of microsomal triglyceride transfer protein gene and manganese superoxide dismutase gene in nonalcoholic steatohepatitis. J Hepatol 40: 781–786
14. Chitturi S, Farrell GC (2001) Etiopathogenesis of nonalcoholic steatohepatitis. Semin Liver Dis 21: 27–41

15. Pessayre D, Mansouri A, Fromenty B (2002) Nonalcoholic steatosis and steatohepatitis. V. Mitochondrial dysfunction in steatohepatitis. Am J Physiol Gastrointest Liver Physiol 282: G193–199
16. Stewart SF, Leathart JB, Chen Y (2002) Valine-alanine manganese superoxide dismutase polymorphism is not associated with alcohol-induced oxidative stress or liver fibrosis. Hepatology 36: 1355–1360

Predictors of Nonalcoholic Steatohepatitis in Japanese Patients: Thioredoxin and NASH

Takeshi Okanoue, Norihito Yamauchi, Masanori Furutani, Akihisa Hirohama, Yoshio Sumida, and Toshiaki Nakashima

Summary. To clarify the biochemical markers to discriminate between nonalcoholic steatohepatitis (NASH) and simple steatosis in Japanese patients and to clarify the clinicopathological features of NASH, we analyzed patients with NASH and simple fatty liver (FL). Seventy-five patients with biopsy-proven NASH and 53 patients with biopsy-proven FL were enrolled. Their clinical characteristics and histological findings were compared. Detection of GB virus (GBV) RNA and SEN virus (SENV) DNA was performed by polymerase chain reaction (PCR). Mutational analysis of the *HFE* gene was performed by PCR-restriction fragment length polymorphism. As a marker of oxidative stress, serum thioredoxin (TRX) levels were determined. Insulin resistance was evaluated by a homeostasis model assessment of insulin resistance (HOMA-IR). Serum TRX levels were significantly elevated in patients with NASH, compared with patients with FL. GBV was detectable in the serum of only one patient with NASH. SEN virus was detected in 50% (15/30) of the patients tested, but the prevalence was not significantly different between the two groups (42% [8/19] in FL and 64% [7/11] in NASH). The *HFE* gene was not detected in any patient. We constructed a receiver operating characteristic (ROC) curve which confirmed that serum TRX and ferritin levels were predictors for distinguishing NASH from FL. HOMA-IR was higher in NASH patients than in FL patients. The pathogenesis of NASH may be associated with insulin resistance and iron-related oxidative stress. The serum TRX level is a parameter for discriminating NASH from simple steatosis.

Key words. Nonalcoholic steatohepatitis, Serum ferritin, Oxidative stress, Thioredoxin, Insulin resistance

Introduction

Nonalcoholic fatty liver disease (NAFLD) is defined as the clinical condition characterized by predominantly macrovesicular steatosis of the liver. It is important to distinguish nonalcoholic steatohepatitis (NASH) from simple fatty liver (FL), because the former can progress to cirrhosis and hepatocellular carcinoma (HCC), while the latter is considered to be a nonprogressive benign disease [1–3]. Although growing evidence

Molecular Gastroenterology and Hepatology, Kyoto Prefectural University of Medicine, Graduate School of Medical Science, Kawaramachi-Hirokoji, Kamigyo-ku, Kyoto 602-8566, Japan supports oxidative stress as the most important factor for the development of NASH, its pathogenic mechanisms are yet to be clearly elucidated [2, 4, 5].

Iron is considered a putative element that interacts with oxygen radicals to induce liver damage and fibrosis [6]. High frequencies of hyperferritinemia and increased hepatic iron stores in NASH have been demonstrated, and an association between *HFE* mutations (C282Y and H63D), hepatic iron overload, and NASH has been suggested [6].

Thioredoxin (TRX) has a variety of biological activities, including the scavenging of active oxygen radicals and the regulation of redox-sensitive molecules. Since TRX is induced by many forms of oxidative stress, serum TRX levels are believed to be a clinically useful indicator of oxidative stress [7, 8].

In most NASH patients, the disease is associated with obesity, hyperlipidemia, and type 2 diabetes mellitus. Thus, it has been considered that insulin resistance plays an important role in the development of NASH.

Certain viruses identified recently have been controversial as to whether infection with such viruses leads to the development of chronic liver disease. GB virus (GBV) was initially suggested as a causative agent of non-A to -E hepatitis, and furthermore as a potential confounder for the progression to NASH [9–11]. TT virus (TTV) was identified from the sera of patients with transfusion-associated hepatitis [12]. There is a possibility that certain TTV genotypes, including genotype 1, influence the development of necrosis, inflammation, and fibrosis of the liver in NAFLD patients [13]. Recently, a novel DNA virus, distantly related to the TTV, was detected in the serum of an intravenous drug abuser also infected with human immunodeficiency virus, and was designated SEN virus (SENV) [14, 15]. Eight different strains have been isolated; SENV-A to -H. Genotypes SENV-D and SENV-H were more prevalent in the serum samples of patients with transfusion-associated non-A to -E hepatitis [16].

There have not been any reports on the association between SENV infection and NAFLD, and very few reports dealing with GBV infection in patients with NAFLD.

Patients, Materials, and Methods

Patients

Seventy-five patients with NASH and 53 patients with FL, diagnosed by liver biopsy, performed at the Department of Gastroenterology and Hepatology, Kyoto Prefectural University of Medicine and related institutions, were enrolled in this study. The degree of obesity was expressed by the body mass index (BMI). A BMI of more than 25 was defined as indicating obesity. Insulin resistance was expressed by homeostasis model assessment for insulin resistance (HOMA-IR). The study protocols were reviewed and approved by the appropriate institutional review boards, and informed consent was obtained from each subject.

Laboratory Data

Serum aspartate aminotransferase (AST), alanine aminotransferase (ALT), gamma glutamyl transpeptidase (GGT), ferritin, total cholesterol (T-Chol), triglyceride (TG), fasting glucose, immunoreactive insulin (IRI), and platelet count (PLT) were determined. Serum TRX levels were examined in some patients.

Liver Histology

Biopsy specimens were stained with hematoxylin and eosin and Masson's trichrome, and with Perls' Prussian blue stain for assessment of iron loading. Steatosis was graded as follows: 1, fewer than 33% of hepatocytes affected; 2, 33%–66% of hepatocytes affected; and 3, more than 66% of hepatocytes affected. Diagnosis of NASH was established by the combined presence of pericentral macrovesicular steatosis, hepatocyte injury and necrosis, mixed inflammatory infiltration, and variable degrees of fibrosis. The degree of inflammation and fibrosis was assessed according to the grading (0 to 3) and staging (0 to 4) system for NASH proposed by Brunt et al. [17]. The degree of iron loading was assessed using a Perls' score of 0 to 4+, based on the scoring system of MacSween et al. [18].

Detection of GBV RNA

Stored serum samples were obtained from 38 subjects, and 30 of these samples were tested for the presence of GBV. Detection of GBV RNA was performed according to the method described by Tan et al. [19].

Detection of SENV DNA

Thirty of the 38 stored serum samples were tested for the presence of SENV-D/H. SENV DNA was determined by PCR, using primers derived from conserved sequences among the SENV strains [14].

Mutational Analyses of the HFE Gene

Twenty-seven of the 75 subjects with NASH were tested for *HFE* C282Y and H63D mutations. Detection of these mutations was performed using PCR and restriction fragment length polymorphism (RFLP), as described previously [20].

Statistical Analysis

We compared continuous variables using the Mann-Whitney *U*-test. The Kruskal-Wallis test was used for multiple group comparisons, and Spearman correlation coefficients were used to examine the relationship between groups. Frequency analysis was performed with the χ^2 test, and with Fisher's exact test especially for 2×2 tables. P values of less than 0.05 were considered significant. To assess the use of clinical parameters in differentiating NASH from simple steatosis, we calculated the sensitivity and specificity for each value of each test and then constructed receiver operating characteristic (ROC) curves.

Results

Patient Demographics and Laboratory Evaluation

The main demographic and clinical laboratory features of patients with FL and NASH are presented in Tables 1 and 2. The sex ratio, BMI, and the prevalences of obesity, type 2 diabetes, and hyperlipidemia did not differ between the two groups. The age was significantly ($P = 0.003$) higher in NASH patients (Table 1). Serum AST levels were found to be significantly ($P < 0.001$) higher in patients with NASH than in patients with FL. Serum ferritin levels in NASH patients were significantly higher ($P < 0.001$) than those in the FL patients, and the frequency of hyperferritinemia was also higher in NASH patients. The PLT levels of NASH patients were significantly ($P = 0.001$) lower than those of FL patients (Table 2).

Comparison of Histological Features Between Simple Steatosis and NASH Patients

The histological features of patients with FL and NASH are presented in Table 3. Hepatic inflammation (grade) and hepatic fibrosis (stage) were rarely seen in FL.

Table 1. Demographics of patients with simple fatty liver and nonalcoholic steatohepatitis (NASH)

	Fatty liver ($n = 53$)	NASH ($n = 75$)	P value
Sex (female)	21/53 (39.6%)	36/75 (48.0%)	0.372
Age (years)	50 (Range, 15–71)	56 (Range, 22–80)	0.003
BMI (kg/m^2)	25.7 (Range, 15.4-35.6)	26.4 (Range, 14.6–42.4)	0.085
Obesity	30/50 (60.0%)	54/74 (73.0%)	0.171
Type 2 diabetes	5/42 (11.9%)	9/63 (14.3%)	0.779
Hyperlipidemia	30/51 (58.8%)	38/70 (54.3%)	0.711

Table 2. Laboratory data of patients with simple fatty liver and NASH

	Fatty liver ($n = 53$)	NASH ($n = 75$)	P value
AST (12–35 IU/l)[a]	41 (12–179)	75 (22–242)	<0.001
ALT (6–33 IU/l)[a]	80 (13–347)	107 (19–316)	0.019
GGT (3–54 IU/l)[a]	90 (19–568)	87 (30–810)	0.777
T-Chol (125–220 mg/dl)[a]	216 (79–313)	205 (149–293)	0.071
TG (31–160 mg/dl)[a]	165 (49–413)	132 (37–879)	0.217
FPG (65–126 mg/dl)[a]	101 (77–280)	102 (83–270)	0.640
HOMA-IR	2.34 (0.91–6.22)*	4.42 (0.53–27.6)**	0.088
Serum ferritin (75–247 ng/ml [M]; 21–75 ng/ml [F])[a]	124 (13–499)	270 (35–1010)	<0.001
Hyperferritinemia	16/45 (35.6%)	54/72 (75.0%)	<0.001
PLT (10.4–34.8 × 10^4/μl)[a]	23.6 (9.7–38.2)	18.6 (6.5–41.0)	0.001

Values in parentheses are ranges, unless indicated otherwise

[a] Normal ranges *; n = 7 **; n = 15

Table 3. Histological findings of patients with simple fatty liver and NASH

	Fatty liver	NASH	*P* value
Steatosis (grade) 1/2/3	14/22/17	31/24/19	0.303
Hepatic inflammation (grade) 0/1/2/3	53/0/0/0	0/39/33/2	<0.001
Hepatic fibrosis (stage) 0/1/2/3/4	51/2/0/0/0	1/29/20/21/3	<0.001
Iron (Perls' score) 0/1/2/3	25/6/5/0	20/25/11/3	0.006

Table 4. Relation between serum thioredoxin (TRX) levels and histological iron score (Perls' score) in patients with NASH and simple steatosis[a]

	Iron score (Perls' score)			*P* value[b]
	0	1	2–3	
NASH ($n = 22$)	40.2 (15.1–69.7)* ($n = 7$)	50.7 (21.5–104.7)** ($n = 9$)	64.6 (18.9–85.3) ($n = 6$)	0.174
Simple steatosis ($n = 13$)	24.6 (16.6–49.8)* ($n = 8$)	30.7 (17.5–34.3)** ($n = 5$)		
Total ($n = 35$)	26.1 (15.1–69.7) ($n = 15$)	35.8 (17.5–104.7) ($n = 14$)	64.6 (18.9–85.3) ($n = 6$)	0.035

* $P = 0.355$ (Mann-Whitney U-test); ** $P = 0.053$ (Mann-Whitney U-test)

[a] Data from patients with Perls' score of 2 or 3 were combined because of the small number of patients

Results are presented as the medians and (ranges) of serum TRX levels

[b] *P* values were calculated by using Spearman correlation analysis

Perls' scores were significantly (P = 0.006) higher in patients with NASH than in patients with FL. Additionally, Perls' scores were found to differ between each histological grade, and they tended to be higher in patients with an advanced grade (Table 4). Higher serum ferritin levels were found in patients with advanced histological grade and in patients with advanced histological stage.

Serum Thioredoxin (TRX) Levels

Serum TRX levels were significantly elevated in patients with NASH (57.7 ng/ml), compared to those in patients with FL (26.8 ng/ml) and those in the controls (23.5 ng/ml; Fig. 1). No difference in the serum TRX levels between sexes were observed for either patient group (NASH patients, $P = 0.805$; FL patients, $P > 0.999$)

ROC curve Analysis for Serum Ferritin and TRX

The ROC curves from serum ferritin and TRX used in discriminating NASH from FL are shown in Fig. 2. The serum ferritin threshold for the prediction of NASH was 124 ng/ml; at this threshold, the sensitivity was 75%, and the specificity was 64.3% (Fig. 2A). On the other hand, the serum TRX threshold was 34.7 ng/ml; at this threshold, the sensitivity was 72.0% and the specificity was 86.7% (Fig. 2B).

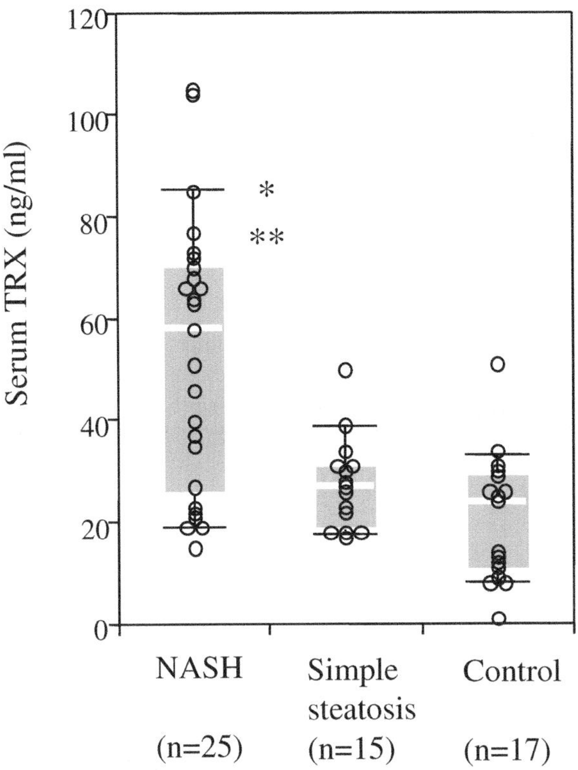

Fig. 1. Serum thioredoxin (*TRX*) levels in patients with nonalcoholic steatohepatitis (*NASH*), those with simple steatosis, and healthy controls. $^{*}P = 0.009$ vs simple steatosis; $^{**}P < 0.001$ vs control.

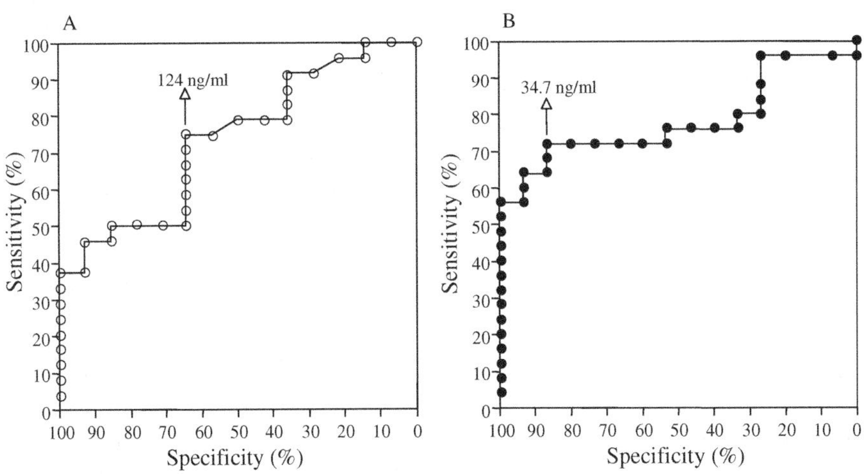

Fig. 2. Receiver operating characteristic (ROC) curves for serum ferritin (**A**) and TRX (**B**) used to discriminate NASH and simple steatosis.

Frequencies of HGV, SENV-D, or SENV-H Infection, and HFE Gene Mutation

Only one patient with NASH was positive for GBV, and none of the patients with FL had HGV. Fifteen of 30 patients whose sera were tested for SEN virus were positive for SENV-D or -H (50%). The prevalence of SENV-D or -H did not significantly differ between FL patients and NASH patients. Neither C282Y mutation nor H63D mutation was observed in the *HFE* genes of any subject.

Discussion

Early studies described NASH mainly in obese, middle aged women, often associated with type 2 diabetes mellitus and hyperlipidemia [3], but the disease is increasingly being recognized in male patients and patients without obesity or diabetes mellitus [1, 2, 21, 22]. BMI values and the prevalence of diabetes mellitus and hyperlipidemia were not significantly different between the patient two groups in the present study.

To the best of our knowledge, no clinical or laboratory parameters have been used to predict NASH that do not require a liver biopsy. The present study demonstrates that serum ferritin and TRX levels were significantly higher in NASH patients than in FL patients. By calculating the area under the ROC curve, we found that the serum ferritin and TRX levels were parameters for discriminating NASH from simple FL [23].

It remains unclear why some patients with NAFLD progress to cirrhosis and others generally have a benign course. Recently, a hypothesis called the 'two-hit process' has been proposed [4]. That is, an aberration in fatty acid and triglyceride metabolism leads to hepatic triglyceride accumulation ('first hit'), and then, a 'second hit' causes progression to NASH. The candidates for this 'second hit' form three categories: factors contributing to oxidative stress and subsequent lipid peroxidation, factors associated with abnormal cytokine production, and factors associated with disordered fatty-acid metabolism and insulin resistance [5]. Iron is considered a putative element that interacts with oxygen radicals in inducing liver damage and fibrosis [6]. High frequencies of hyperferritinemia and increased hepatic iron stores in NASH have been demonstrated [6, 22]. Furthermore, a significantly high prevalence of *HFE* mutations in patients with NASH was reported as a factor responsible for liver fibrosis via increasing hepatic iron deposition [6], but recent studies have failed to confirm this [24, 25]. There were no patients with *HFE* mutations in the present study, in agreement with a previous report indicating that the frequencies of *HFE* mutations in the Japanese population are low (C282Y, 0%; and H63D, 0.99%) [26]. Thus, hyperferritinemia and hepatic iron deposition seem to be characteristic conditions for NASH in Japan.

We examined whether infection by GBV and the newly discovered human virus, SEN virus, had any influence on the histological features of NAFLD. We found that the frequencies of GBV infection and SENV-D/-H infection did not significantly differ between the two patient groups. Our results suggest that neither GBV infection nor SENV infection are involved in the development and progression of NAFLD.

The most common abnormality in liver function tests of NAFLD is a two- to fivefold elevation in serum aminotransferase level [1–3]. The AST/ALT ratio is reported to be less than 1 in most instances. When the AST/ALT ratio is more than 1, it suggests that there is an advanced form of NAFLD [1,21,22]. In the present study, the median values of the serum aminotransferase levels in the two groups were mildly elevated, but the serum AST level was significantly higher in NASH patients than in FL patients. A higher serum AST level suggests the existence of severe hepatocyte injury.

Hyperlipidemia has been reported to be commonly observed in NAFLD [1,21,22, 24]. Several studies indicated that there was no significant difference in the serum lipid state between FL and NASH [21, 23, 27]. In our series, the serum T-Chol level was significantly lower in NASH patients than in FL patients. Commonly, a low T-Chol level in patients with cirrhosis is considered to be connected with a decline in liver synthesis ability [28].

In conclusion, the increases in serum TRX levels and hepatic iron concentrations suggest that iron-induced oxidative stress may play an important role in the pathogenesis of NASH. The serum TRX level can help to discriminate NASH from simple FL, and may be a predictor of the disease severity in patients with NASH. It is not confirmed that *HFE* mutation is involved in the development of NASH in Japan. There are insufficient data to confirm a causal role for GBV and SENV infections in NASH.

References

1. Sanyal AJ (2002) Technical review on nonalcoholic fatty liver disease. Gastroenterology 123: 1705–1725
2. Younossi ZM, Diehl AM, Ong JP (2002) Nonalcoholic fatty liver disease: an agenda for clinical research. Hepatology 35: 746–752
3. Powell EE, Cooksley WGE, Hanson R, Searle J (1990) The natural history of nonalcoholic steatohepatitis: a follow-up study of 42 patients for up to 21 years. Hepatology 11: 74–80
4. Day CP, James OFW (1998) Steatohepatitis: a tale of two 'hits'? Gastroenterology 114: 842–845
5. James O, Day C (1999) Non-alcoholic steatohepatitis: another disease of affluence. Lancet 353: 1634–1636
6. George DK, Goldwurm S, Macdonald GA (1998) Increased hepatic iron concentration in nonalcoholic steatohepatitis is associated with increased fibrosis. Gastroenterology 114: 311–318
7. Hirota K, Matsui M, Iwata S (1997) AP-1 transcription activity is regulated by a direct association between thioredoxin and Ref-1. Proc Natl Acad Sci USA 94: 3633–3638
8. Nakamura H, Nakamura K, Yodoi J (1997) Redox regulation of cellular activation. Annu Rev Immunol 15: 351–369
9. Linnen J, Wages J Jr, Zhang-Keck ZY (1996) Molecular cloning and disease association of hepatitis G virus: a transfusion-transmissible agent. Science 271: 505–508
10. Simons JN, Leary TP, Dawson GJ (1995) Isolation of novel virus-like sequences associated with human hepatitis. Nat Med 1: 564–569
11. Kiyosawa K (1997) Non-alcoholic steatohepatitis and GB virus-C/hepatitis G virus infection: is there a causal relationship? Intern Med 36: 236–237
12. Nishizawa T, Okamoto H, Konishi K (1997) A novel DNA virus (TTV) associated with elevated transaminase levels in posttransfusion hepatitis of unknown etiology. Biochem Biophys Res Commun 241: 92–97
13. Tokita H, Murai S, Kamitsukasa H (2001) Influence of TT virus on the histopathological features of nonalcoholic fatty liver disease. Hepatol Res 19: 197–211

14. Primi D, Fiordalisi G, Mantero JL, Identification of SENV genotypes. International patent number WO0028039 (international application published under the patent cooperation treaty). http://ep.espacenet.com
15. Tanaka Y, Primi D, Wang RYH (2001) Genomic and molecular evolutionary analysis of a newly identified infectious agent (SEN virus) and its relationship to the TT virus family. J Infect Dis 183: 359–367
16. Umemura T, Yeo AET, Sottini A (2001) SEN virus infection and its relationship to transfusion-associated hepatitis. Hepatology 33: 1303–1311
17. Brunt EM, Janney CG, DiBisceglie AM (2000) Nonalcoholic steatohepatitis: a proposal for grading and staging the histologic lesions. Am J Gastroenterol 94: 2467–2474
18. MacSween RNM, Anthony PP, Sheuer PJ (1987) Pathology of the liver. Churchill Livingstone, Edinburgh, p 185
19. Tan D, Matsumoto A, Conry-Cantilena C (1999) Analysis of hepatitis G virus (HGV) RNA, antibody to HGV envelope protein, and risk factors for blood donors coinfected with HGV and hepatitis C virus. J Infect Dis 179: 1055–1061
20. Kazemi-Shirazi L, Datz C, Maier-Dobersberger T (1998) The relation of iron status and hemochromatosis gene mutations in patients with chronic hepatitis C. Gastroenterology 116: 127–134
21. Matteoni CA, Younossi ZM, Gramlich T (1999) Nonalcoholic fatty liver disease: a spectrum of clinical and pathological severity. Gastroenterology 116: 1413–1419
22. Bacon BR, Farahvash MJ, Janney CG (1994) Nonalcoholic steatohepatitis: an expanded clinical entity. Gastroenterology 107: 1103–1109
23. Sumida Y, Nakashima T, Yoh T (2003) Serum thioredoxin levels as a predictor of steatohepatitis in patients with nonalcoholic fatty liver disease. J Hepatol 38: 32–38
24. Angulo P, Keach J, Batts K (1999) Independent predictors of liver fibrosis in patients with nonalcoholic steatohepatitis. Hepatology 30: 1356–1362
25. Mendler M, Turlin B, Moirand R (1999) Insulin resistance-associated hepatic iron overload. Gastroenterology 117: 1155–1163
26. Sohda T, Yanai J, Soejima H (1999) Frequencies in the Japanese population of HFE gene mutations. Biochem Genet 37: 63–68
27. Loguercio C, Girolamo V, Sio IF (2001) Non-alcoholic fatty liver disease in an area of southern Italy: main clinical, histological, and pathophysiological aspects. J Hepatol 35: 568–574
28. Powell EE, Kroon PA (1992) Liver, lipoproteins and disease: II. Clinical relevance of disordered cholesterol metabolism in liver disease. J Gastroenterol Hepatol 7: 225–231

Clinical Features of Patients with Nonalcoholic Fatty Liver Disease

Etsuko Hashimoto, Hiroyuki Kaneda, Yoko Yoshioka, Makiko Taniai, Katsutoshi Tokushige, and Keiko Shiratori

Summary. We assessed the clinicopathological features of nonalcoholic fatty liver disease (NAFLD) in patients stratified by the stage of fibrosis. One-hundred and ninety-three patients were diagnosed as having NAFLD at Tokyo Women's Medical University or an affiliated hospital, from 1990 to September 2003, and their clinical data were collected prospectively. The diagnosis of NAFLD was based on the following criteria: (1) the presence of steatosis (affecting >30% of hepatocytes) or steatohepatitis, with steatohepatitis being defined by detection of steatosis (affecting >10% of hepatocytes), inflammatory infiltrates, and ballooning degeneration with or without Mallory bodies, pericellular fibrosis, and perivenular fibrosis; (2) intake of less than 20 g of ethanol per week; and (3) appropriate exclusion of other liver diseases. We assessed the clinicopathological features of NAFLD in patients stratified by the stage of fibrosis. The median age of the patients was 53 years, with a range of 10 to 83 years. There were 96 males and 97 females. Eighty-five percent of the patients had at least one of the features of the metabolic syndrome. Histologically, 29 patients had established cirrhosis. In regard to severe fibrosis, females and older patients were more common. There were correlations between serum hyaluronic acid level, type IV collagen level, or platelet count and the stage of fibrosis. Eight patients developed hepatocellular carcinoma. Except for 1 F3 patient, they all had cirrhosis. Liver biopsy is invasive, expensive, and not suitable for all NALFD patients. Because we found correlations between serum fibrosis markers, or platelet count and the stage of fibrosis, these markers may be useful to identify NASH with severe fibrosis among NAFLD patients.

Key words. Nonalcoholic steatohepatitis, Nonalcoholic fatty liver disease, Liver cirrhosis, Hepatocellular carcinoma, Steatohepatitis

Introduction

Nonalcoholic steatohepatitis (NASH) is a clinicopathological entity characterized by the development of hepatic histological changes, resembling those induced by excessive alcohol intake, that occur in the absence of alcohol abuse [1]. NASH is generally

Institute of Gastroenterology, Tokyo Women's Medical University, 8-1 Kawada-cho, Shinjuku-ku, Tokyo 162-8666, Japan considered to be a mild condition, but it can sometimes progress rapidly or cause cirrhosis, and may even lead to the development of hepatocellular carcinoma (HCC) [1–14]. Cirrhosis is present in 2% to 28% of patients at diagnosis, so NASH shows a wide range of histology, from minimal fibrosis to cirrhosis.

The category of nonalcoholic fatty liver disease (NAFLD) includes both simple fatty liver and NASH, but the difference between NASH and fatty liver remains unsettled because there is significant diversity of opinion among expert pathologists regarding the specific features of NASH [15, 16]. Generally, fibrosis is the most important pathological change that occurs in liver disease. Accordingly, stratification of NAFLD by the severity of fibrosis seems to be a reasonable method of analyzing the clinicopathological features of NASH.

Patients

One hundred and ninety-three patients were diagnosed as having NAFLD at Tokyo Women's Medical University or an affiliated hospital from 1990 to September 2003, and their clinical data were collected prospectively. Informed consent was obtained from each patient, and the study protocol conformed to the ethical guidelines of the 1975 Declaration of Helsininki. The diagnosis of NAFLD was based on the following criteria: (1) The presence of steatosis (affecting >30% of hepatocytes) or steatohepatitis, with steatohepatitis being defined by the detection of steatosis (affecting >10% of hepatocytes), inflammatory infiltrates, and ballooning degeneration with or without Mallory bodies, pericellular fibrosis, and perivenular fibrosis; (2) intake of less than 20 g of ethanol per week, as confirmed by the attending physician and family members who were in close contact with the patient; and (3) appropriate exclusion of other liver diseases, such as alcoholic liver disease, viral hepatitis, autoimmune hepatitis, drug-induced liver disease, primary biliary cirrhosis, primary sclerosing cholangitis, biliary obstruction, and metabolic liver diseases [15, 16]. To rule out viral hepatitis, patients were excluded if they were positive for hepatitis B surface antigen (HBsAg), antibody to hepatitis C virus (anti-HCV), or hepatitis C RNA (HCV-RNA) by the polymerase chain reaction. No patient had a history of jejunoileal bypass surgery.

Obesity was defined by a body mass index (BMI) of more than 25, according to the Japanese Obesity Association. The diagnosis of type II diabetes mellitus was based on Japanese criteria (random blood glucose >200 mg/dl, or fasting glucose >126 mg/dl, or hemoglobin A_{1c} >6.5% on two occasions). Hyperlipidemia was diagnosed on the basis of treatment with lipid-lowering medication or raised total cholesterol and/or triglyceride levels on at least two occasions. Hypertension was diagnosed if patients were on antihypertensive therapy or the blood pressure was 140/90 mm Hg or more. None of the patients received drug treatment for NASH before liver biopsy. A complete history was obtained and physical examination was performed in all patients. Hepatomegaly was diagnosed by ultrasonography.

Methods

All patients underwent measurement of the following laboratory parameters: liver function tests (aspartate aminotransferase [AST], alanine aminotransferase [ALT], total bilirubin, alkaline phosphatase [ALP], gamma-glutamyltranspeptidase [GGTP]);

total protein; albumin; prothrombin time; hepaplastin test; platelet count; hepatitis B serology (HBsAg; antibody to hepatitis B surface antigen (anti-HBs), and antibody to hepatitis B core antigen [anti-HBc]); hepatitis C serology (anti-HCV and HCV-RNA); triglycerides; total cholesterol; autoantibodies (antinuclear antibodies, anti-smooth muscle antibody, and antimitochondrial antibody); immunoglobulins; iron profile (iron, ferritin, and total iron-binding capacity); type IV collagen; hyaluronic acid; protein induced by vitamin K absence-II, by enzyme immunoassay; and alpha-fetoprotein, by enzyme immunoassay.

Liver Histology

All liver biopsy specimens were examined using the following stains: hematoxylin-eosin, Mallory, silver reticulin, Victoria blue stain for copper-binding protein, and Perls iron stain. Assessment was done by one reviewer (E.H.) without knowledge of the clinical and biochemical data of the patients. Fibrosis was scored using a five-grade scale: F0, normal connective tissue; F1, foci of pericellular fibrosis in zone 3; F2, perivenular or pericellular fibrosis confined to zones 3 and 2, with or without portal/periportal fibrosis; F3, bridging or septal fibrosis; and F4, cirrhosis [15–17]. Steatosis was graded on a scale of 1 to 3: 1, mild (affecting 10%–29% of hepatocytes); 2, moderate (30%–69% of hepatocytes); and 3, severe (>70% of hepatocytes). After evaluation of ballooning degeneration, Mallory bodies, giant mitochondria, disarray of hepatocytes, lobular inflammation, focal necrosis, Councilman bodies, lipogranulomas, pigmented macrophages, and lipogranulomas, a grade of mild, moderate, or severe inflammation was assigned based on the reviewer's overall impression.

Results

The median age of the patients was 53 years, with a range of 10 to 83 years. There were 96 males and 97 females, so both sexes were equally represented.

The age distribution for each sex is shown in Fig. 1. Males showed two peak ages, the thirties and the fifties, while the female age distribution had a single peak, in the fifties to sixties. The only difference in risk factors for NASH between men and women in their twenties and thirties was a higher prevalence of hyperlipidemia and obesity in men.

Eighty-nine patients (46%) were detected on the basis of abnormal liver function tests during annual health checks and 85 (44%) were detected during follow-up for other diseases. In 19 patients (10%), abnormal liver function was detected after they presented with fatigue and/or abdominal distension ($n = 12$), jaundice ($n = 4$), hepatic coma ($n = 1$), or hematemesis due to variceal bleeding ($n = 2$).

The demographic and laboratory data of the NAFLD patients are summarized in Table 1. Eighty-five percent of the patients had at least one of the features of the metabolic syndrome. The median AST level was 52 IU/l and the median ALT level was 77 IU/l.

Histologically, 10 patients had no fibrosis, while 71 were classified as having F1, 37 as F2, 46 as F3 (bridging fibrosis), and 29 as established cirrhosis (Table 2). There were 43 patients with mild steatosis, while 63 showed moderate steatosis, and 87 had severe

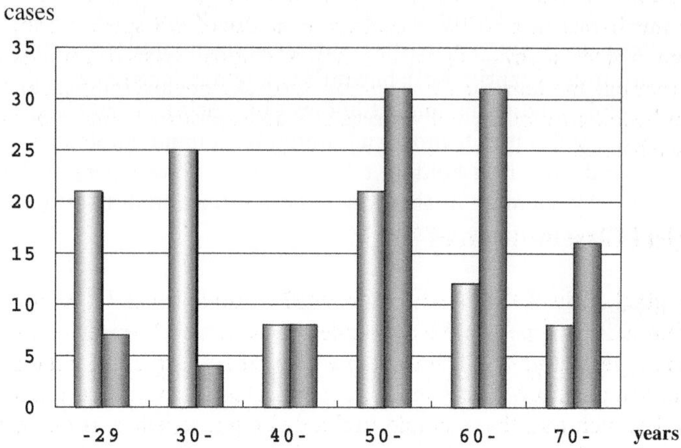

Fig. 1. Age distribution by sex (male, *light bars*, $n = 96$; female, *dark bars*, $n = 97$). Male age distribution peaked twice, in the thirties and the fifties. Female age distribution peaked once, in the fifties to sixties.

Table 1. Demographic and laboratory data ($n = 193$)

Type 2 diabetes mellitus	75 (39%)
Obesity	131 (68%)
Hyperlipidemia	104 (54%)
Hypertension	54 (28%)
Without metabolic syndrome	29 (15%)
AST	9–392 IU/l (52 IU/l)
ALT	5–740 IU/l (77 IU/l)
γGTP	10–487 IU/l (67 IU/l)
T-Bil.	0.2–2.8 mg/dl (0.6 mg/dl)
Platelet count	6–45 × 10^4/μl (22.7 × 10^4/μl)

Figures in parentheses are median values, unless otherwise indicated

Table 2. Liver histology ($n = 193$)

Fibrosis	F0	10 (5%)
	F1	71 (37%)
	F2	37 (19%)
	F3	46 (24%)
	F4	29 (15%)
Steatosis	Mild	43 (22%)
	Moderate	63 (33%)
	Severe	87 (45%)
Inflammation	Mild	70 (36%)
	Moderate	108 (56%)
	Severe	15 (8%)

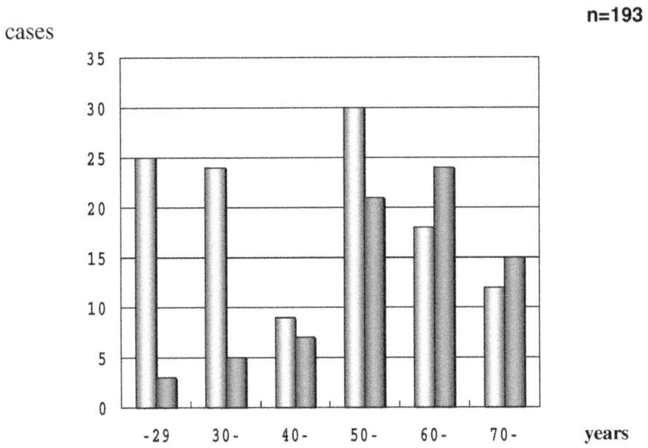

Fig. 2. Age distribution by fibrosis (mild, F0–2, *light bars*; severe, F3–4, *dark bars*). For patients up to their thirties, mild fibrosis was much more common than severe fibrosis. On the other hand, severe fibrosis was more common in older patients.

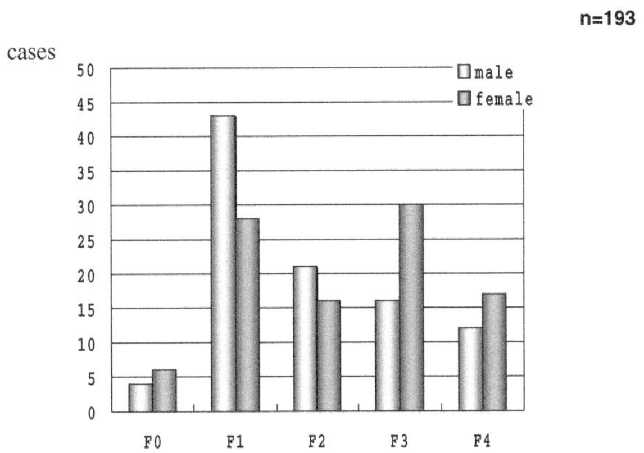

Fig. 3. Sex distribution for each fibrosis stage. In F1–2, the prevalence of males was higher than females. However, in severe fibrosis (F3–4), the prevalence of females was higher.

steatosis. Inflammatory changes were mild in 70 patients, moderate in 108, and severe in 15.

Figure 2 shows the age distribution of severe and mild fibrosis. In patients up to their thirties, mild fibrosis was much more common than severe fibrosis. Conversely, severe fibrosis was more common than mild fibrosis in the older patients. Concerning the sex distribution in each stage of fibrosis, males were more common than females in F1 and F2. In severe fibrosis (F3 or F4), however, females were more common (Fig. 3). The increased prevalence of women and elderly subjects among patients with severe fibrosis suggests that female sex and aging may be risk factors for progression.

The laboratory parameters for each stage of fibrosis are shown in Fig. 4. Transaminase levels were highest in F3. Concerning the AST/ALT ratio, ALT levels were higher than AST levels before the onset of cirrhosis, and the ratio was less than 1.0, while AST levels were higher after cirrhosis developed. The platelet count was significantly decreased after the onset of cirrhosis. In contrast, GGTP and iron parameters were similar at each stage of fibrosis. Albumin and prothrombin time were slightly decreased in the cirrhotic stage. Concerning serum markers of fibrosis, the type IV

Fig. 4. Distribution of laboratory data for each fibrosis stage. *AST*, aspartate aminotransferase; *ALT*, alanine aminotransferase; *γ-GTP*, gamma-glutamyltranspeptidase; *PT*, prothrombin time.

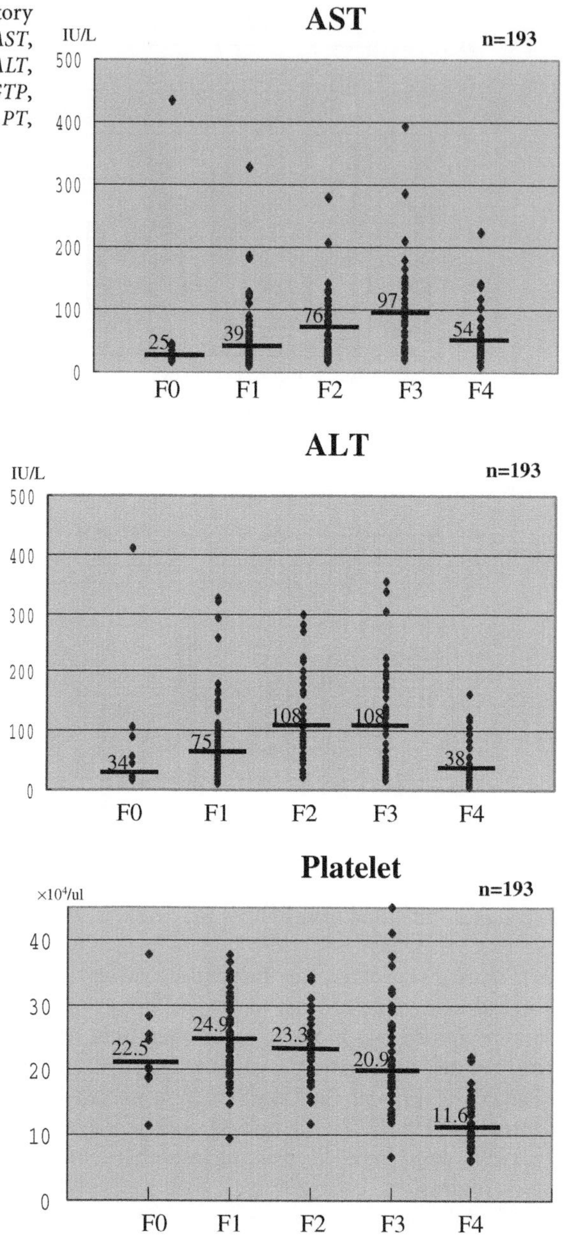

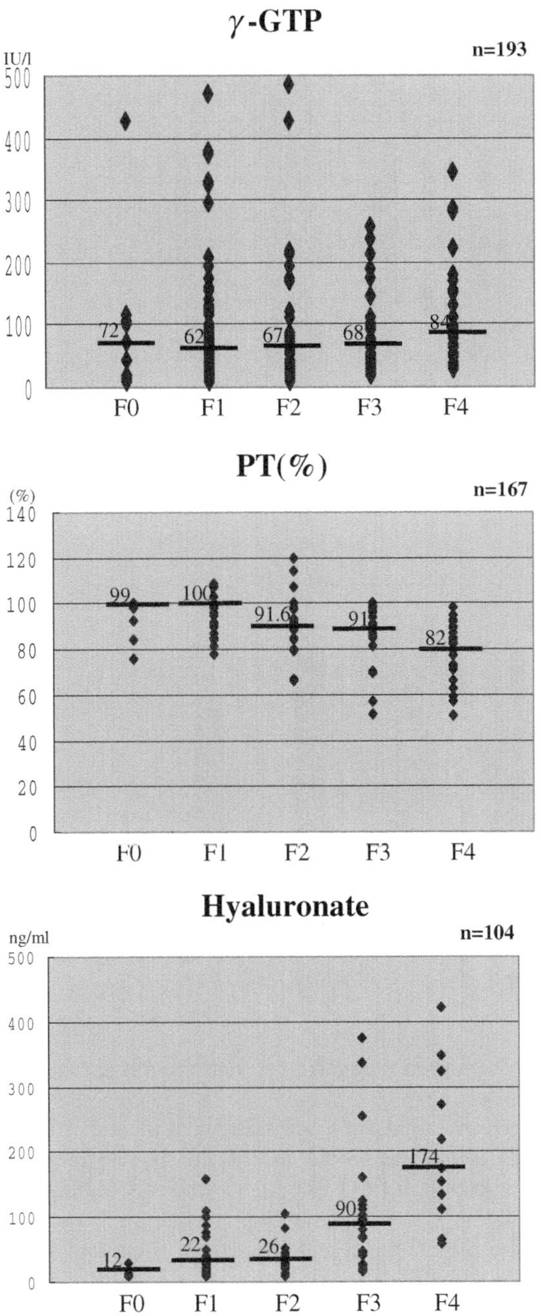

Fig. 4. *Continued*

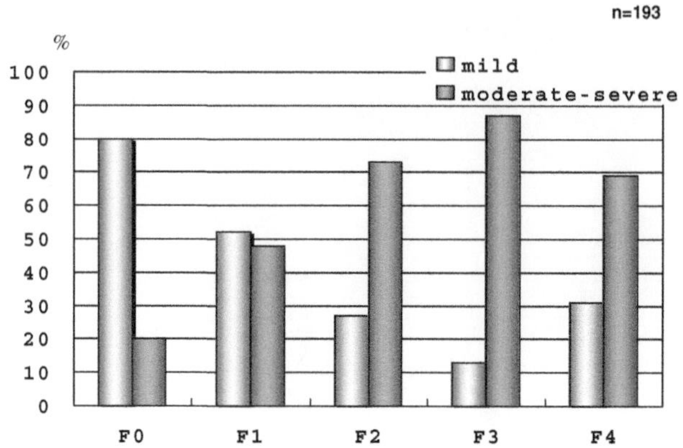

Fig. 5. Distribution of necroinflammatory changes for each fibrosis stage. The prevalence of moderate to severe necroinflammatory changes was higher in patients with advancing fibrosis.

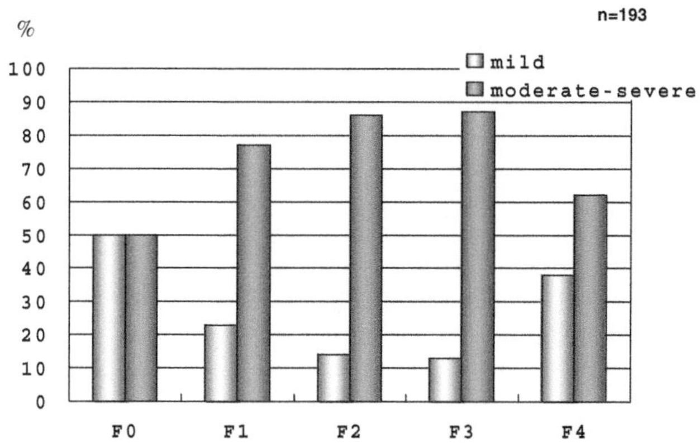

Fig. 6. Distribution of steatosis for each fibrosis stage. The frequency of moderate to severe steatosis was higher in F1 to F3, while this frequency was decreased in F4.

collagen and hyaluronic acid levels showed a positive correlation with the stage of fibrosis.

Histologically moderate to severe inflammatory infiltrates were increased in the patients with severe fibrosis, the difference was not significant (Fig. 5). The frequency of moderate to severe steatosis was higher in F1 to F3 patients, and was decreased in the patients with cirrhosis (Fig. 6).

NASH was associated with cirrhosis in 12 males and 17 females. Their median age was 66 years, with a range of 16 to 83 years. Hospital admission was for gastrointestinal varices in 8 patients, to evaluate hepatic tumors in 6, because of hepatic coma in 1, and for assessment of liver dysfunction in the others. Two patients with no pertinent medical history developed sudden variceal bleeding before the diagnosis of NASH. On admission, 4 patients had jaundice and 1 had hepatic coma. Twenty-two patients

Table 3. Clinical features of patients with NASH and HCC

	Age (years)	Sex	Obesity	DM	HL	HT	AST (IU/l)	ALT (IU/l)	Platelets ($10^4/\mu l$)
1.	56	M		○			44	43	18
2.	64	F		○		○	33	40	8.8
3.	64	M	○	○	○	○	34	55	21
4.	68	F					39	29	6.8
5.	69	F	○	○	○		57	38	9.8
6.	71	F	○	○		○	39	31	16
7.	72	M	○				39	22	8.5
8.	77	F	○			○	55	29	17

	HBsAg	Anti-HBs	Anti-HBc	Anti-HBc × 200	Anti-HCV	HCV-RNA
1.	–	–	–	–	–	–
2.	–	–	–	–	–	–
3.	–	+	+	–	–	–
4.	–	–	–	–	–	–
5.	–	–	–	–	–	–
6.	–	–	–	–	–	–
7.	–	–	–	–	–	–
8.	–	–	–	–	–	–

underwent gastrointestinal fiberscopy, and 15 of them had esophageal varices (68%). Three patients developed HCC during follow-up of cirrhotic NASH, 3 patients were simultaneously diagnosed as having NASH and HCC, and 2 HCC patients were retrospectively diagnosed as having NASH by review of surgical specimens of the noncancerous liver (which showed typical steatohepatitis).

Table 3 shows the clinical features of our patients with NASH and HCC (3 males and 5 females). They were aged from 56 to 77 years. All except one patient had features of the metabolic syndrome. AST and ALT levels were less than twice the upper limit of normal in all patients and the platelet counts ranged from 6.8 to 21 × 10^5/ml. One patient was weakly positive for anti-HBc and anti-HBs, but the others showed no hepatitis virus markers. The patient with weakly positive anti-HBc and anti-HBs had no histological features of hepatitis B, such as portal inflammation or 'ground-glass' hepatocytes. Seven patients had cirrhosis and one had F3 fibrosis, but the grades of steatosis, inflammation, and ballooning degeneration varied among the patients (Table 4).

Discussion

We assessed the clinicopathological features of NAFLD in patients stratified by the stage of fibrosis. Most of the NAFLD patients were asymptomatic, with mild elevation of transaminases, and 85% had at least one of the symptoms of metabolic syndrome. The increased prevalence of women and older patients with NAFLD among those with more advanced fibrosis suggested that female sex and older age may be risk factors for progression.

Table 4. Histological features of livers with NASH and HCC

	Fibrosis	Inflammation	Steatosis	Mallory body	Ballooning	Hemoside-rosis
1.	F4	Mod	Mod	◎	Severe	−
2.	F4	Mod	Severe	◎	Mod	−
3.	F4	Mod	Mod	◎	Mod	−
4.	F3	Mod	Mod	◎	Mod	+
5.	F4	Mod	Mod	◎	Severe	−
6.	F4	Mild	Mod	◎	Severe	−
7.	F4	Mod	Mod	◎	Mod	−
8.	F4	Mild	Mild	○	Mod	−

Mod; moderate

Although fatty liver is readily detected by noninvasive imaging, liver biopsy is necessary for a diagnosis of NASH, because imaging does not detect fibrosis or inflammation, especially in the presence of fat [18]. However, liver biopsy is invasive, expensive, and not suitable for all NAFLD patients [16]. Because we found correlations between the serum hyaluronic acid level, type IV collagen level, or platelet count and the stage of fibrosis, these serum markers may be useful to identify NASH with severe fibrosis among NAFLD patients.

The AST/ALT ratio is almost always less than 1 in NASH patients, except after the onset of cirrhosis [5, 19]. This is not the case with alcoholic liver disease, so the AST/ALT ratio can be useful to distinguish alcoholic steatohepatitis from NASH.

Conflicting data have been reported about the contribution of iron to liver damage in NASH patients [1, 5, 20]. We did not find any relationship between serum iron parameters and the stage of fibrosis, and mild iron deposition was only seen in 14 patients (7%).

In our study, 15% of the NAFLD patients showed cirrhosis on their first biopsy and eight patients developed HCC. Most cirrhotic NASH was asymptomatic and the patients showed mild elevation of transaminases with relatively well-preserved liver function (albumin, ammonia, and prothrombin time), elevated serum fibrosis markers, and a low platelet count. The incidence of gastrointestinal varices was high (68%), and two patients suffered from hematemesis before the diagnosis of liver disease. However, during almost 3 years of follow-up, no patient died of cirrhosis. On the other hand, four patients died of HCC.

The most important etiological factors for HCC are hepatitis B and C virus infection. We analyzed hepatitis virus infection by serological methods only, and found one HCC patient who was positive for anti-HBs and anti-HBc, but this patient had no histological features of chronic hepatitis B. Hence, we concluded that hepatitis B virus infection did not play a role in the development of HCC associated with NASH. Several other reports have already described the development of HCC in patients with NASH or obesity-related cryptogenic cirrhosis [9–14].

In summary, NAFLD is emerging as one of the most common liver diseases in Japan because of increasing obesity. Patients with cirrhotic NASH may develop HCC, and this occurs often enough to warrant regular screening.

References

1. Ludwig J, Viggiano TR, McGill DB, Ott BJ (1980) Nonalcoholic steatohepatitis. Mayo Clinic experiences with a hitherto unnamed disease. Mayo Clin Proc 55: 434–438
2. Powel EE, W. Cooksley WGE, Hanson R, Searle J, Halliday JW, Powell LW (1990) The natural history of steatohepatitis: a follow-up study of 42 patients for up to 21 years. Hepatology 11: 74–80
3. Matteoni CA, Younossi ZM, Gramlich T (1999) Nonalcoholic fatty liver disease: a spectrum of clinical and pathological severity. Gastroenterology 116: 1413–1419
4. Willner IR, Waters B, Patil SR, Reuben A, Morelli J, Riely CA (2001) Ninety patients with nonalcoholic steatohepatitis: insulin resistance, familial tendency, and severity of disease. Am J Gastroenterol 96: 2957–2961
5. Angulo P, Keach JC, Batts KP, Lindor KD (1999) Risk factors of liver fibrosis in patients with nonalcoholic steatohepatitis. Hepatology 30: 1356–1362
6. Shimada M, Hashimoto E, Kaneda H, Noguchi S, Hayashi N (2002) Nonalcoholic steatohepatitis: risk factors for liver fibrosis. Hepatol Res 24: 429–438
7. Caldwell SH, Hespenheide EE (2002) Subacute liver failure in obese women. Am J Gastroenterol 97: 2058–2062
8. Kuwabara H, Hoshii Y, Mori H (2003) Nonalcoholic steatohepatitis-related cirrhosis with subacute liver failure; an autopsy case. Dig Dis Science 48: 1669–1670
9. Shimada M, Hashimoto E, Taniai M (2002) Hepatocellular carcinoma in patients with non-alcoholic steatohepatitis. J Hepatol 37: 154–160
10. Zen Y, Katayanagi K, Tsunyama K, Harada K, Araki I, Nakanuma Y (2001) Hepatocellular carcinoma arising in non-alcoholic steatohepatitis. Pathol Int 51: 127–131
11. Cotrim HP, Parana R, Braga E, Lyra L (2000) Nonalcoholic steatohepatitis and hepatocellular carcinoma: natural history? Am J Gastroenterol 95: 3018–3019
12. Bugianesi E, Leone N, Vanni E, Marchesini G, Brunello F, Carucci P, Musso A, Paolis PD, Capussotti L, Salizzoni M, Rizzetto M (2002) Expanding the natural history of NASH: from cryptogenic cirrhosis to hepatocellular carcinoma. Gastroenterology 123: 134–140
13. Marrero JA, Fontana R, Su GL, Conjeevaram HS, Emick DM, Lok AS (2002) NAFLD may be a common underlying liver disease in patients with hepatocellular carcinoma in the United States. Hepatology 36: 1349–1354
14. Ratziu V, Bonyhay L, Di Martino V, Charlotte F, Cavallaro L, Sayegh-Taiturier MH, Giral P, Grimaldi A, Opolon P, Poynard T (2002) Survival, liver failure, and hepatocellular carcinoma in obesity-related cryptogenic cirrhosis. Hepatology 35: 1485–1493
15. Neuschwander-Tetri BA, Caldwell SH (2003) Nonalcoholic steatohepatitis: Summary of an AASLD single topic conference. Hepatology 37: 1202–1219
16. Sanyal AJ (2002) AGA technical review on nonalcoholic fatty liver disease. Gastroenterology 123: 1705–1725
17. Brunt EM, Janney CG, Di Bisceglie AM (1999) Nonalcoholic steato-hepatitis: a proposal for grading and staging the histological lesions. Am J Gastroenterol 94: 2467–2474
18. Saadeh S, Younossi ZM, Remer EM, Gramlich T, Ong JP, Hurley M, Mullen KD, Cooper JN (2002) The utility of radiological imaging in nonalcoholic fatty liver disease. Gastroenterology 123: 745–750
19. Sheth SG, Flamm SL, Gordon FD, Chopra S (1998) AST/ALT ratio predicts cirrhosis in patients with chronic hepatitis C virus infection. Am J Gastroenterol 93: 44–48
20. Chitturi S, Weltman M, Farrell GC (2002) HFE mutations, hepatic iron, and fibrosis: ethnic-specific association of NASH with C282Y but not with fibrotic severity. Hepatology 36: 142–149

Pathogenesis and Significance of Restricted Diet and Exercise Therapy in Nonalcoholic Steatohepatitis (NASH)

TAKATO UENO[1], TORU NAKAMURA[2], NOZOMI SASAKI[3], YASUYO MORITA[3], EISUKE NAGATA[3], and MICHIO SATA[2]

Summary. The risk factors that are most strongly associated with nonalcoholic fatty liver disease (NAFLD) are: age greater than 40 to 50 years, and severe obesity, diabetes mellitus (DM), or hyperlipidemia (especially hypertriglyceridemia). The pathogenesis of nonalcoholic steatohepatitis (NASH) is multifactorial. Insulin resistance, fatty acids, and oxidant stress may be important pathogenic factors in NASH. Efforts are presently underway to define the role of these factors and to determine whether modifying them (for example, by improving insulin sensitivity) could be effective in the treatment of the condition. At present, lifestyle changes involving exercise and dietary restrictions appear to be an effective means of improving NASH. Physicians should actively check for the presence of NAFLD in those who are overweight and who have diabetes mellitus. The treatment is usually directed toward optimizing body weight. The role of pharmacological agents remains to be established, and much more work is necessary to define the pathogenesis of NASH and to develop effective treatments.

Key words. Nonalcoholic fatty liver disease (NAFLD), Nonalcoholic steatohepatitis (NASH), Insulin receptor substance 1 (IRS-1), Leptin, Restricted diet and exercise therapy

Introduction

Nonalcoholic fatty liver disease (NAFLD) is currently defined as fat accumulation in the liver exceeding 5%–10% by weight, but it is evaluated in terms of the percentage of fat-laden hepatocytes observed by light microscopy. In NAFLD, an age greater than 40 to 50 years and severe obesity, diabetes mellitus (DM), or hyperlipidemia (especially hypertriglyceridemia) are the most reliable risk factors [1]. When the fat content in the liver is above 10%, fat droplets begin to appear in many hepatocytes. By the time the amount of fat exceeds 30% of the liver weight, almost all of the hepatocytes contain a large drop of fat. In addition, the degree of NAFLD correlates with increased body weight [2]. Some investigators have reported that NAFLD progresses to liver cirrhosis [3–7] or to hepatocellular carcinoma [8, 9].

[1] Research Center for Innovative Cancer Therapy, Kurume University, 67 Asahi-machi, Kurume, Fukuoka 830-0011, Japan
[2] Second Department of Internal Medicine, Kurume University School of Medicine, 67 Asahi-machi, Kurume, Fukuoka 830-0011, Japan
[3] Nagata Hospital, 523-1 Shimomiyanaga-machi, Yanagawa, Fukuoka 832-0059, Japan

On the other hand, the development of steatosis, steatohepatitis, progressive hepatic fibrosis, and cirrhosis is most likely the result of multiple metabolic abnormalities, such as insulin resistance, oxidant stress, fatty acids, and inflammatory cytokines [1].

In this chapter, we would like to review the significance of NAFLD, and we will discuss the management of nonalcoholic steatohepatitis (NASH), including restricted diet and exercise therapy, in relation to the pathogenesis of NAFLD.

Pathogenesis and Complications of NAFLD

Insulin Resistance

Insulin resistance is common in patients with NAFLD and NASH. Insulin modulates intracellular signaling through the tyrosine kinase activity of the insulin receptor. A major mechanism regulating insulin receptor substance-1 (IRS-1) signaling involves excess free fatty acids (FFAs). FFAs impair the tyrosine phosphorylation of IRS-1 [10]. Insulin sensitivity is also regulated by peptide mediators. In the normal human liver, IRS-1 is mainly localized in hepatocytes (Fig. 1a). Adipose tissue, especially mesenteric fat with its venous blood flowing directly to the liver, is a rich source of cytokine and peptide hormone production that regulates downstream metabolic activity. These

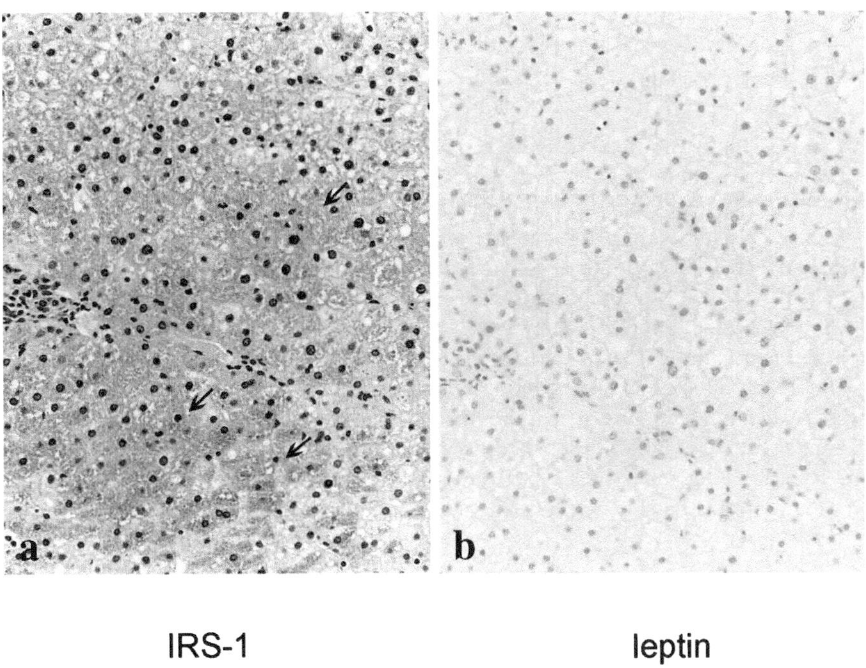

Fig. 1a,b. Immunolocalization of **a** insulin and **b** leptin receptor substance-1 (*IRS-1*) in normal liver tissues. The immunoreactive products of leptin are very scarce in the normal liver, but those of IRS-1 are mainly localized in the hepatocytes (*arrows*). × 100.

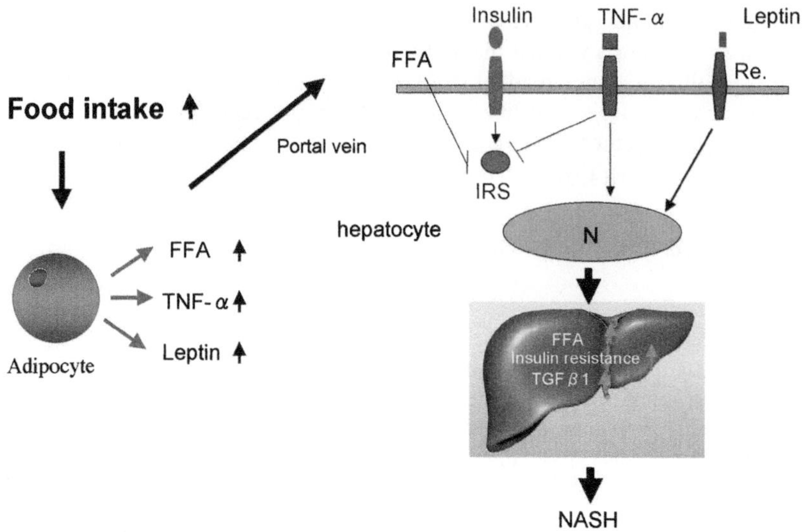

Fig. 2. Overeating and nonalcoholic steatohepatitis (*NASH*). With an increase of food intake, agents containing free fatty acid (*FFA*), tumor necrosis factor-α (*TNF-α*), and leptin are overproduced by adipocytes, and arrive at the liver by way of the portal vein. In the liver, IRS-1 is influenced by FFA, TNF-α, and other agents. The expression and function of IRS-1 appears to be suppressed. On the other hand, leptin seems to be upregulated. Eventually the liver metabolism is disturbed and NASH may occur. *N*, nucleus; *Re.*, receptor; *TGFβ1*, transforming growth factor β1.

agents include tumor necrosis factor-α (TNF-α), leptin, adiponectin, and plasminogen activator inhibitor-1 [1] (Fig. 2).

TNF-α knockout mice fail to develop insulin resistance after induction of obesity [11]. TNF-α appears to stimulate the serine phosphorylation of IRS-1, and I kappa B kinase β (IKK β) may play an important role in this process.

Leptin may also be important in regulating the partitioning of fat between mitochondrial β-oxidation and triglyceride synthesis. In the normal human liver, very little leptin is present (Fig. 1b). Defects in leptin signaling are associated with the preferential accumulation of fat and impaired β-oxidation of fat in the liver. In NASH, it was suggested that leptin is necessary for the development of fibrosis [12, 13]. On the other hand, Chitturi et al. [14] reported that circulating leptin in patients with NASH correlated with hepatic steatosis, but not with hepatic fibrosis.

Adiponectin has a cytokine structure and appears to improve hepatocyte insulin sensitivity.

Oxidant Stress

Oxidant stress is frequently stated to be a central mechanism of hepatocellular injury in NASH. Multiple possible sources of oxidant stress in NAFLD have been identified, and include cytochrome P450, peroxisomal β-oxidation, mitochondrial electron leak, and recruited inflammatory cells.

Treatment of NAFLD

The treatment of NAFLD, including NASH, includes modification of the clinical conditions associated with NAFLD, such as type II DM, hyperlipidemia, and obesity. Specific therapeutic interventions tested so far include weight reduction, and the use of ursodeoxycholic acid (UDCA), clofibrate, troglitazone, vitamin E, and other agents.

Exercise Therapy and Restricted Diet

Those who are overweight (body mass index [BMI] >25 kg/m^2) and have NAFLD should be considered for a weight-loss program (Figs. 3, 4). A target of 10% of baseline weight is often used as an initial weight-loss goal. Dietary recommendations generally include both caloric restrictions and a decrease in saturated fats, as well as a proportion of total fats of 30% or less of the total calories. Both intermittent and daily exercise can help achieve weight loss and improve insulin sensitivity.

We previously reported that patients with NAFLD (including NASH and fatty liver [FL]) who were subjected to dietary restriction and an exercise regimen (Fig. 3) lost weight for 3 months, and achieved a significant improvement in their serum transaminase levels compared with those before treatment (Figs. 4, 6). In addition, serial liver biopsy results (degrees of steatosis and fibrosis) in these patients showed a significant improvement after treatment (Figs. 4, 7). Moreover, in regard to BMI, steatosis, and ballooning of hepatocytes, the FL group had improved compared with the NASH group after treatment (Fig. 5).

Subjects with a BMI of more than 35 kg/m^2 and NAFLD may be considered for more aggressive weight management, including a gastric bypass. However, patients should

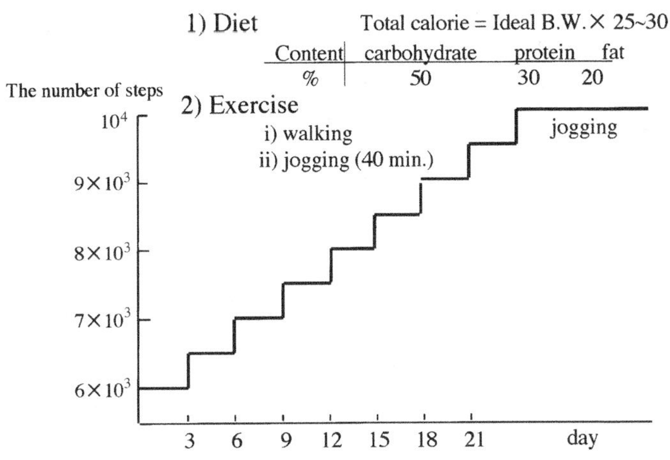

Fig. 3. Therapeutic plan for patients with nonalcoholic liver disease (NAFLD): diet and exercise. A diet that consists of total ideal body weight (*B.W.*) times 25 to 30 calories per day is designed. For exercise, a program of walking is established, in which the subject walks 1000 steps the first week. This is increased by 1000 steps per week until 10 000 steps are reached, after which jogging for 40 min is started.

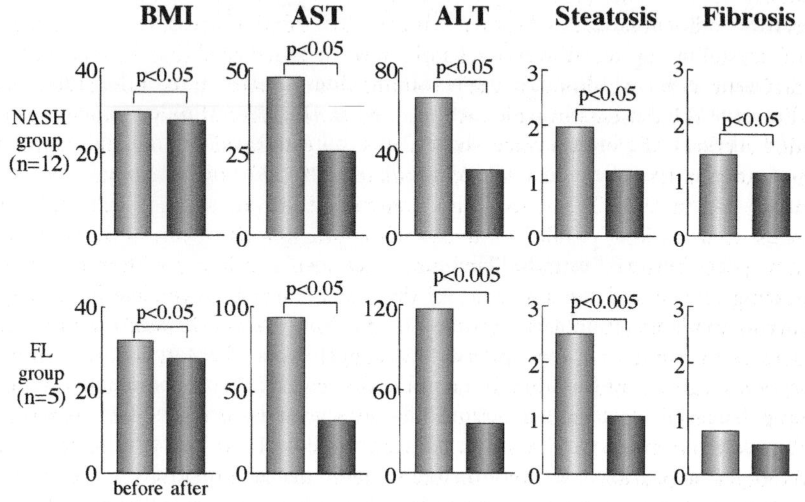

Fig. 4. Comparison of body mass index (*BMI*), aspartate aminotransferase (*AST*), and alanine aminotransferase (*ALT*) levels, and histological findings before and after treatment in NASH and fatty liver (*FL*) groups. BMI, AST, and ALT levels after treatment in the NASH and FL groups were significantly decreased compared with the levels before treatment. In addition, the degrees of steatosis and fibrosis after treatment in the NASH and FL groups tended to decrease compared with those before treatment.

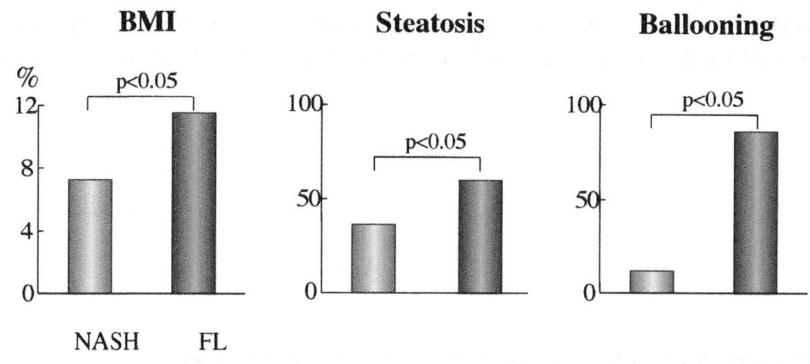

Fig. 5. Comparison of improvement rate between NASH and FL groups. The values for BMI, steatosis, and ballooning hepatocytes in the FL group were significantly improved compared with those in the NASH group.

be monitored for signs of subacute nonalcoholic steatohepatitis during weight loss, and liver function should be checked at appropriate intervals, depending on the rapidity of the weight loss.

Pharmacological Treatment

In addition to obesity, hyperlipidemia is seen in 20% to 81% of patients with NASH [5, 15, 16]. Studies of treatment strategies aimed at alleviating hyperlipidemia in

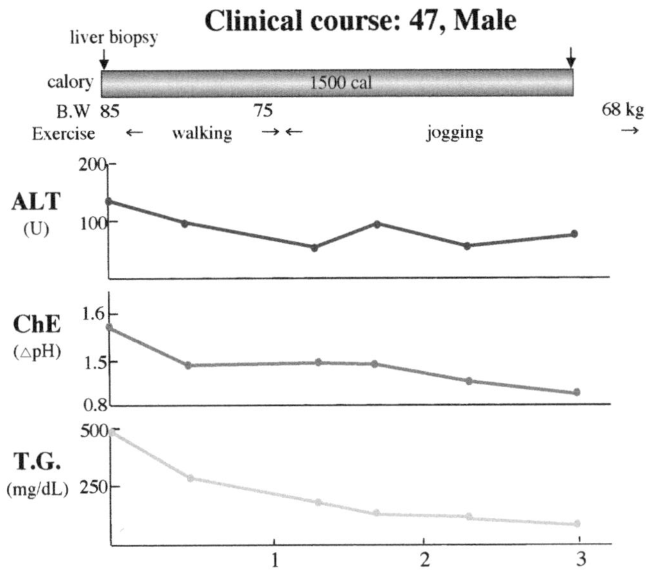

Fig. 6. Clinical course of restricted diet and exercise therapy in a patient with NASH (47-year-old man). Body weight, *ALT*, cholinesterase (*ChE*), and triglyceride (*T.G.*) levels were gradually improved by the treatment.

patients with NASH have had conflicting results [17–20]. In one study, 16 patients with hypertriglyceridemia and NASH were treated with clofibrate for 12 months [17]. There were no significant changes in biochemical or histologic parameters. The only randomized controlled trial of lipid-lowering agents in the treatment of NASH examined 46 patients who were randomized to receive either gemfibrozil or no therapy, regardless of serum triglyceride levels [17]. There was a significant decrease in serum transaminases, but histologic data were unavailable [17]. As reported previously, these conditions are part of the spectrum of clinical manifestations of the insulin-resistance syndrome. Therefore, agents that improve insulin sensitivity may be of particular value in the treatment of NASH. Marchesini et al. [18] have recently reported a pilot study of 14 patients with NAFLD who were given metformin 500 mg three times a day for 4 months. Although no sequential biopsies were available, significant improvements in the aminotransferase levels were noted [18]. An open-label study of troglitazone, a peroxisome-proliferator activated receptor γ (PPAR-γ) agonist that improves insulin sensitivity, showed a significant decrease in liver volume, as measured on magnetic resonance imaging, in patients with lipoatrophic diabetes, severe insulin resistance, and NAFLD [19]. Caldwell et al. [20] treated 10 patients with biopsy-proven NASH with troglitazone for 6 months. At the end of the treatment period, serum aminotransferase levels were normalized in 7 of the 10 patients; however, this biochemical improvement was accompanied by only a minimal improvement in histology on serial liver biopsies [20].

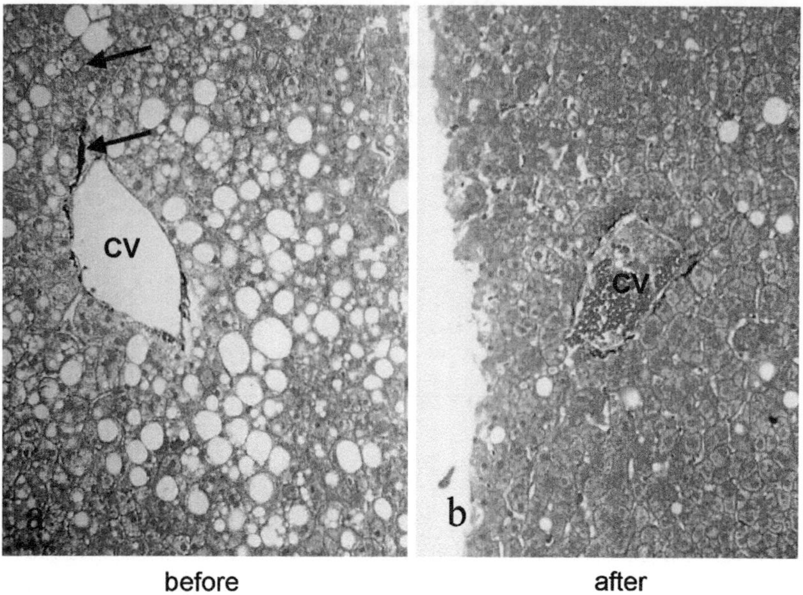

Fig. 7a,b. Light micrographs showing liver specimens before and after therapy in the patient with NASH whose clinical course is shown in Fig. 6. Steatosis and perivenular fibrosis (*arrows*) improved after treatment. *CV*, central vein. × 400.

Conclusions

NAFLD is frequently associated with the presence of obesity, insulin resistance, and hyperlipidemia. There is increasing evidence that NASH, part of the spectrum of NAFLD, can progress to cirrhosis and hepatocellular carcinoma. Physicians should actively check for the presence of NAFLD in those who are overweight and have DM. The treatment is usually directed toward optimizing body weight. The role of pharmacological agents remains to be established, and much more work is necessary to define the pathogenesis of NASH and to develop effective treatment modalities.

References

1. Neuschwander-Tetri BA, Caldwell SH (2003) Nonalcoholic steatohepatitis: summary of an AASLD single topic conference. Hepatology 37: 1202–1219
2. Dixon JB, Bhathal PS, O'Brien PE (2001) Nonalcoholic fatty liver disease: predictors of nonalcoholic steatohepatitis and liver fibrosis in the severely obese. Gastroenterology 121: 91–100
3. Adler M, Schaffner F (1979) Fatty liver hepatitis and cirrhosis in obese patients. Am J Med 67: 811–816
4. Ito S, Tsukada Y, Motomura Y, Ichinoe A (1979) Five patients with nonalcoholic diabetic cirrhosis. Acta Hepatogastroenterol 26: 90–97

5. Ludwig J, Viggiano TR, McGill DB, Oh BJ (1980) Nonalcoholic steatohepatitis: Mayo Clinic experiences with a hitherto unnamed disease. Mayo Clin Proc 55: 434–438
6. Caldwell SH, Oelsner DH, Iezzoni JC, Hespenheide EE, Battle EH, Driscoll CJ (1999) Cryptogenic cirrhosis: clinical characterization and risk factors for underlying disease. Hepatology 29: 664–669
7. Struben VM, Hespenheide EE, Caldwell SH (2000) Nonalcoholic steatohepatitis and cryptogenic cirrhosis within kindreds. Am J Med 108: 9–13
8. Bugianesi E, Leone N, Vanni E, Marchesini G, Brunello F, Carucci P, Musso A, DePaolis P, Capussotti L, Salizzoni M, Rizzetto M (2002) Expanding the natural history of nonalcoholic steatohepatitis: from cryptogenic cirrhosis to hepatocellular carcinoma. Gastroenterology 123: 134–140
9. Shimada M, Hashimoto E, Taniai M, Hasegawa K, Okuda H, Hayashi N, Takasaki K, Ludwig J (2002) Hepatocellular carcinoma in patients with non-alcoholic steatohepatitis. J Hepatol 37: 154–160
10. Saltiel AR (2001) New perspectives into the molecular pathogenesis and treatment of type 2 diabetes. Cell 104: 517–529
11. Uysal KT, Wiesbrock SM, Marino MW, Hotamisligil GS (1997) Protection from obesity-induced insulin resistance in mice lacking TNF-α function. Nature 389: 610–614
12. Ikejima K, Takei Y, Honda H, Hirose M, Yoshikawa M, Zhang YJ, Lang T, Fukuda T, Yamashina S, Kitamura T, Sato N (2002) Leptin receptor-mediated signaling regulates hepatic fibrogenesis and remodeling of extracellular matrix in the rat. Gastroenterology 122: 1399–1410
13. Saxena NK, Ikeda K, Rockey DC, Frieman SL, Anania FA (2002) Leptin in hepatic fibrosis: evidence for increased collagen production in stellate cells and lean littermates of ob/ob mice. Hepatology 35: 762–771
14. Chitturi S, Farrell G, Frost L, Kriketos A, Lin R, Fung C, Liddle C, Samarasinghe D, George J (2002) Serum leptin in NASH correlates with hepatic steatosis but not fibrosis: a manifestation of lipotoxicity? Hepatology 36: 403–409
15. Diehl AM, Goodman Z, Ishak KG (1988) Alcohol like liver disease in nonalcoholics. A clinical and histologic comparison with alcohol-induced liver injury. Gastroenterology 95: 1056–1062
16. Matteoni CA, Younossi ZM, Gramlich T, Boparai N, Liu YC, McCullough AJ (1999) Nonalcoholic fatty liver disease: a spectrum of clinical and pathological severity. Gastroenterology 116: 1413–1419
17. Basaranoglu M, Acbay O, Sonsuz A (1999) A controlled trial of gemfibrozil in the treatment of patients with nonalcoholic steatohepatitis. J Hepatol 31: 384
18. Marchesini G, Brizi M, Bianchi G, Tomassetti S, Zoli M, Melchionda N (2001) Metformin in non-alcoholic steatohepatitis. Lancet 358: 893–894
19. Arioglu E, Duncan-Morin J, Sebring N, Rother KI, Gottlieb N, Lieberman J, Herion D, Kleiner DE, Reynolds J, Premkumar A, Sumner AE, Hoofnagle J, Reitman ML, Taylor SI (2000) Efficacy and safety of troglitazone in the treatment of lipodystrophy syndromes. Ann Intern Med 133: 263–274
20. Caldwell SH, Hespenheide EE, Redick JA, Iezzoni JC, Battle EH, Sheppard BL (2001) A pilot study of a thiazolidinedione, troglitazone, in nonalcoholic steatohepatitis. Am J Gastroenterol 96: 519–525

Mammalian Target of Rapamycin (mTOR)

Kazuyoshi Yonezawa[1,2]

Summary. The mammalian target of rapamycin (mTOR) is a giant serine/threonine protein kinase that plays a crucial role in a nutrient-sensitive signaling pathway that regulates cell growth and proliferation. The activity of mTOR is controlled by amino acids (especially by leucine, one of the branched-chain amino acids), in addition to growth factors and overall energy supply through an AMP-activated protein kinase. mTOR, in complex with two other proteins, raptor and mLST8, phosphorylates p70 S6 kinase and eukaryotic initiation factor 4E (eIF4E) binding protein to regulate mRNA translation. The signaling pathway upstream of mTOR involves the protein products of the genes mutated in tuberous sclerosis (*TSC1* and *TSC2*) and the small GTPase, Rheb, whose overexpression rescues mTOR from inactivation in vivo by amino-acid withdrawal. In this review, we describe recent progress in the understanding of the molecular mechanisms of rapamycin action through mTOR.

Key words. Rapamycin, mTOR, Raptor, Amino acids, Translation

Introduction

The potent immunosuppressive drugs FK506 (tacrolimus) and rapamycin (sirolimus) interfere with signal transduction pathways required for T-cell activation and growth. The distinct inhibitory effects of these drugs on the T-cell activation program are mediated through the formation of pharmacologically active complexes with members of a family of intracellular receptors termed the FK506 binding proteins (FKBPs). The FKBP12/FK506 complex specifically binds to and inhibits calcineurin, a signaling protein required for transcriptional activation of the interleukin-2 gene in response to T-cell antigen receptor engagement. Rapamycin exhibits its pharmacological effects through molecular mechanisms that are completely distinct from those of FK506. Here recent progress in the understanding of the molecular mechanisms of rapamycin action will be reviewed.

[1] Biosignal Research Center, Kobe University, 1-1, Rokkodai-cho, Nada-ku, Kobe 657-8501, Japan
[2] CREST, Japan Science and Technology Agency, 4-1-8 Honmachi, Kawaguchi, Saitama 332-0012, Japan

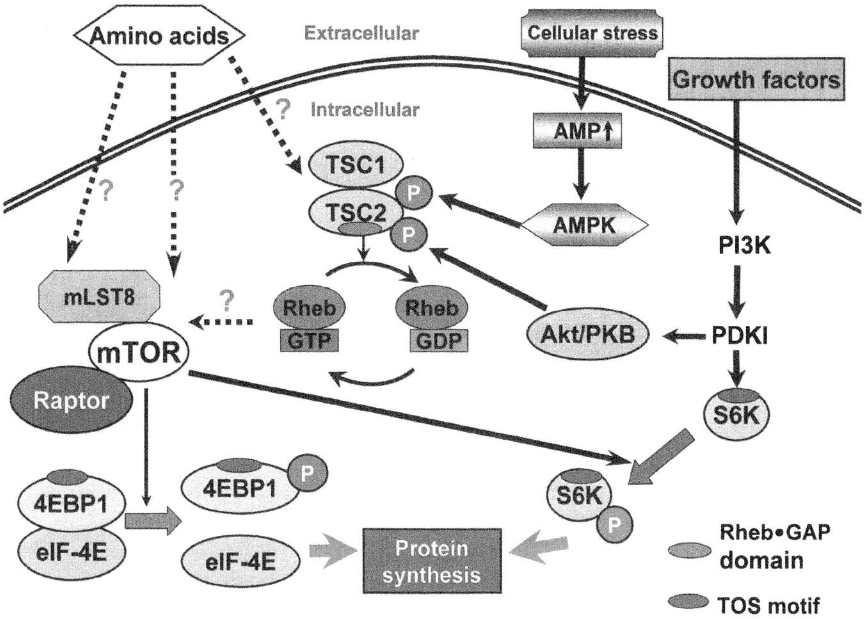

Fig. 1. A model of the mammalian target of rapamycin (*mTOR*) signaling pathway. Amino acids (especially, leucine) and growth factor-inputs regulate the mTOR signaling pathway. Growth factor-dependent Akt/PKB activation, through PI3K and 3-phosphoinositide-dependent protein kinase-1 (*PDK1*), crosstalks with the stimulation of the mTOR-dependent response through the tuberous sclerosis complex (*TSC*) proteins, TSC1 and TSC2, which serve as negative regulators of the mTOR pathway. The small guanosine triphosphatase (GTPase), Rheb, appears to be a direct target of TSC2's intrinsic GTPase-activating function. Rheb-guanosine triphosphate (*GTP*) appears to be a positive modulator of mTOR signaling. Raptor serves as a scaffolding protein that binds p70 S6 kinase (*p70S6k*; *S6k*) and eukaryotic initiation factor 4E (*eIF4E*) binding protein 1 (*4EBP1*) through their TOR signaling (*TOS*) motifs, and raptor facilitates phosphorylation by mTOR. mLST8 binds constitutively with the kinase domain of mTOR. Under conditions of cellular stress resulting in elevations of cellular AMP, the AMP-activated protein kinase (*AMPK*)-catalyzed phosphorylation of TSC2 appears to enhance the ability of the TSC1/TSC2 complex to inhibit mTOR. *GAP*, GTPase-activating protein; *GDP*, guanosine diphosphate.

Discovery of Rapamycin and In Vivo Pharmacological Actions

The bacterial macrolide rapamycin was identified during antibiotic screening. Rapamycin was isolated from a strain of *Streptomyces hygroscopicus* derived from a soil sample collected from the Vai Atore region of Easter Island (Rapa Nui) [1]. Rapamycin is now used as an immunosuppressant to prevent graft rejection after transplantation. In addition, a recent clinical trial has demonstrated great efficacy of a rapamycin-eluting stent in preventing restenosis of coronary arteries after angioplasty. Furthermore, rapamycin and two analogues, CCI-779 and RAD001, are promising anticancer drugs, potently inhibiting a wide range of human tumor cell lines [2].

The Target of Rapamycin (TOR)

Studies in yeast, in which two independent groups first identified the target of the FKBP/rapamycin complex, have made enormous contributions to our understanding of the mechanism of rapamycin action in mammalian cells. The extreme growth-sensitivity of *Saccharomyces cerevisiae* to rapamycin allowed for the selection of rapamycin-resistant mutants that identified genes mediating rapamycin sensitivity. The mutant alleles of two genes (*TOR1* and *TOR2*) were found to confer resistance to growth inhibition by rapamycin [3]. TOR is a highly conserved giant protein and its mammalian ortholog is known as mammalian TOR (mTOR; also known as FRAP, RAFT1, or RAPT). The human *mTOR* gene encodes a protein of 2549 amino acids. mTOR contains a kinase domain near the C-terminus, most closely related to the phosphatidylinositol 3-kinase (PI3K)-related kinase family, which includes ATM, ATR, and DNA-PK kinases. However, mTOR functions as a serine/threonine protein kinase [2]. Other characteristic structures include N-terminal HEAT repeats, the FAT/FATC domains surrounding the kinase domain, and the FKBP-rapamycin binding (FRB) domain. Rapamycin complexed with FKBP12 binds the TOR polypeptide through the FRB domain and inhibits signaling by TOR [3].

mTOR Functions

A major function of TOR in all cells is mRNA translation [4]; in mammalian cells, mTOR stimulates translational initiation through the phosphorylation of eukaryotic initiation factor 4E (eIF4E) binding protein 1 (4E-BP1). 4E-BP1 binds to eIF4E (a 7-methyl-guanosine mRNA cap-binding protein) and prevents eIF4E from binding to the scaffold protein eIF4G, thereby inhibiting the formation of the active translational complex, eIF4F [4]. Insulin or mitogens stimulate the phosphorylation of 4E-BP1, resulting in the dissociation and disinhibition of eIF-4E, enabling recruitment of the latter into the eIF-4F complex [4]. mTOR also directly phosphorylates and, in collaboration with 3-phosphoinositide-dependent protein kinase-1 (PDK1), activates p70 S6 kinase (p70S6k) [5]; the latter regulates cell size [6] through incompletely defined mechanisms [7, 8] and also phosphorylates 40S ribosomal protein S6. p70S6k is proposed to play an important role in the translation of a subclass of mRNAs that contain a short oligopyrimidine sequence [9], although this has been disputed recently [10]. Several studies of *Drosophila melanogaster* TOR have demonstrated that TOR proteins play a critical role in controlling cell growth by regulating several translational effectors in response to the nutritional environment [11–13].

Upstream Inputs to Regulate TOR Activity

As to the regulation of TOR activity, TOR in *S. cerevisiae* (*Sc*TOR) appears to be responsive primarily to nutrient sufficiency; rapamycin or the deletion of both *Sc*TOR genes elicits cell-cycle arrest in G0 and a phenotype resembling that of nutrient depletion [3]. In mammalian cells, mTOR output is sensitive to nutrient (especially amino acid) sufficiency, but is also controlled by overall energy supply through AMP-activated protein kinase (AMPK) and by inputs from cell surface receptors through the PI3K-AKT/PKB pathway [14].

In mammals, in concert with other amino acids, leucine, one of the branched chain amino acids, has been reported to be the primary indicator of amino-acid supply for controlling mTOR activity [15, 16]. Abundant leucine increases mTOR activity, both in animals and in various cell types in culture, including hepatocytes [2]. Leucine appears not to use upstream signaling elements in insulin and growth-factor pathways. Just how leucine increases mTOR kinase activity has not yet been elucidated, although there is evidence implicating changes in mitochondrial metabolism [17].

AMPK is the mammalian ortholog of Snf1 [18, 19] and exists as a heterotrimeric complex comprising a catalytic α subunit and noncatalytic β and γ subunits [18, 19]. Under conditions of hypoxia, exercise, ischemia, heat shock, and low glucose, AMPK is activated allosterically by rising cellular AMP and by phosphorylation of the catalytic α subunit by one or more AMPK kinases on Thr-172, located in the 'T-loop' of the catalytic domain [18, 19]. Once activated, AMPK phosphorylates multiple downstream substrates aimed at conserving existing ATP levels. AMPK reduces further ATP expenditure by inhibiting key enzymes in biosynthetic pathways such as acetyl-CoA carboxylase in fatty acid synthesis and 3-hydroxy-3-methyl-CoA reductase in cholesterol synthesis [18]. AMPK also increases the supply of ATP; for example, by stimulating the rate of fatty acid oxidation and cellular glucose uptake [18].

Modulation of AMPK activities using various reagents, including 5-aminoimidazole-4-carboxamide ribonucleoside (AICAR), D-glucose and its analogues, and mutant AMPK subunits, affects the activity and phosphorylation state of p70S6k, indicating convergence of AMPK signaling and mTOR/amino-acid signaling pathways [20].

mTOR-Interacting Proteins

Recent findings have confirmed that mTOR functions as part of a larger signaling complex. The functional mTOR complex is comprised of mTOR in association with the proteins raptor [21, 22] (KOG1 in *S. cerevisiae* [23]) and mLST8 [23] (also called GβL [24]). The ability of the mTOR kinase to phosphorylate these (and presumably other) targets is heavily dependent on the association of mTOR with raptor, inasmuch as raptor binds the mTOR substrates 4E-BP and p70S6k and presents them to mTOR [21]. In fact, mTOR is completely unable to phosphorylate 4E-BP in vitro in the absence of raptor, or in vivo if 4E-BP is mutated in the 'TOS' motif [25], the 4E-BP segment that mediates binding to raptor [26–29]. The ability of mTOR to regulate p70S6k is also strongly dependent on the association of p70S6k with raptor; mutation of the p70S6k TOS motif reduces mTOR-catalyzed phosphorylation of p70S6k in vitro by approximately 75% and renders p70S6k insensitive to inhibition in vivo by rapamycin or to regulation by ambient amino acids [25]. Our recent observations indicate that rapamycin inhibits mTOR function, at least in part, by inhibiting the interaction of raptor with mTOR; this action uncouples mTOR from its substrates, and inhibits mTOR signaling without altering mTOR's intrinsic catalytic activity [30]. mLST8 [23, 24] is a 36-kDa polypeptide whose predicted structure is composed entirely of seven WD repeats, presumably arrayed in a so-called 'beta propeller' [31].

mLST8 plays a necessary but incompletely defined role in mTOR regulation; the polypeptide binds tightly to the mTOR catalytic domain and enhances the association of raptor with mTOR [24]; however, other roles remain unknown.

Tuberous Sclerosis Complex (TSC1/TSC2) and Rheb

Although the mechanisms by which nutrient and mitogenic inputs control mTOR activity are incompletely understood, recent evidence indicates that the tuberous sclerosis complex (TSC1/TSC2) is a negative regulator acting upstream of mTOR and a major target through which AKT/PKB, AMPK, and perhaps amino-acid sufficiency control mTOR activity [2, 32–34]. TSC1 and TSC2 function together as an obligatory heterodimer; loss of either polypeptide results in an essentially identical phenotype at the organismal or cellular level. A complete loss of TSC function in humans results in the development of hamartomas, benign tumors composed of multiple dysplastic cell types [32]. In *Drosophila*, loss-of-function (LOF) mutations of either TSC1 or TSC2 have growth-promoting effects that are dominant over LOF mutations in the insulin receptor, PI3K or AKT/PKB, but are suppressed by inactivation of TOR or p70S6k [33]. Biochemical studies in mammalian cells have established that inactivation of TSC results in the constitutive activation of p70S6k, which is resistant to inhibition by withdrawal of amino acids, but sensitive to inhibition by rapamycin [32, 34]. Notably, AKT/PKB, whose overexpression indirectly promotes the hyperphosphorylation of 4E-BP and activation of p70S6k, phosphorylates TSC2 at several sites and may accelerate the degradation of both TSC2 and TSC1, perhaps by promoting the dissociation of the heterodimer [35–37]. In contrast, AMPK-catalyzed phosphorylation of TSC2 enhances the ability of the TSC1/TSC2 complex to inhibit TOR [38]. Thus, the TSC complex is a potent negative regulator of TOR signaling and at least one locus of PI3K/AKT, energy, and perhaps amino-acid regulation [39] of the TOR pathway.

As to the mechanisms by which the TSC complex regulates TOR signaling, Gao and coworkers [39] detected a direct interaction between recombinant TSC1/2 and TOR during transient expression. Moreover, several groups have recently reported that the small GTPase Rheb is a positive regulator of growth in *Drosophila*, epistatic to the TSC complex, but requires TOR to achieve growth stimulation [40–43]. Subsequent work has established that *Drosophila* and mammalian TSC2, both of which contain a C-terminal GTPase-activator (GAP) domain, directly stimulate Rheb GTPase in vitro [38, 41, 44–46]. The effectors utilized by Rheb to control cell function are as yet unknown. Rheb is most closely related in amino-acid sequence to the Ras subfamily of small guanosine triphosphatase (GTPases).

Whether TSC1/2 and/or Rheb bind(s) to the mTOR complex containing raptor and whether mLST8 modulates the signaling function and kinase activity of mTOR remain important but unanswered questions. Further investigation should offer new insights into the regulation of the mTOR signaling pathway in response to the nutritional environment.

Acknowledgment. The work by the author discussed in this commentary was supported in part by research grants from the Ministry of Education, Culture, Sports, Science, and Technology of Japan.

References

1. Abraham RT, Wiederrecht GJ (1996) Immunopharmacology of rapamycin. Annu Rev Immunol 14: 483–510
2. Harris TE, Lawrence JCJ (2003) TOR signaling. Sci STKE 212: re15
3. Jacinto E, Hall M (2003) Tor signalling in bugs, brain and brawn. Nat Rev Mol Cell Biol 4: 117–126
4. Gingras AC, Raught B, Sonenberg N (2001) Regulation of translational initiation by FRAP/mTOR. Genes Dev 15: 807–826
5. Isotani S, Hara K, Tokunaga C, Inoue H, Avruch J, Yonezawa K (1999) Immunopurified mammalian target of rapamycin phosphorylates and activates p70 S6 kinase alpha in vitro. J Biol Chem 274: 34493–34498
6. Kozma SC, Thomas G (2002) Regulation of cell size in growth, development and human disease: PI3K, PKB and S6K. Bioessays 2: 65–71
7. Stolovich M, Tang H, Hornstein E, Levy G, Cohen R, Bae S, Birnbaum MJ, Meyuhas O (2002) Transduction of growth or mitogenic signals into translational activation of TOP mRNAs is fully reliant on the phosphatidylinositol 3-kinase-mediated pathway but requires neither S6K1 nor rpS6 phosphorylation. Mol Cell Biol 22: 8101–8113
8. Hannan KM, Brandenberger Y, Jenkins A, Sharkey K, Cavanaugh A, Rothblum LI, Poortinga G, McArthur GA, Pearson RB, Hannan RD (2003) mTOR-dependent regulation of ribosomal gene transcription requires S6K1 and is mediated by phosphorylation of the carboxy-terminal activation domain of the nucleolar transcription factor UBF. Mol Cell Biol 23: 8862–8877
9. Jefferies HB, Fumagalli S, Dennis PB, Reinhard C, Pearson RB, Thomas G (1997) Rapamycin suppresses 5′TOP mRNA translation through inhibition of p70s6k. EMBO J 16: 3693–3704
10. Tang H, Hornstein E, Stolovich M, Levy G, Livingstone M, Templeton D, Avruch J, Meyuhas O (2001) Amino acid-induced translation of TOP mRNAs is fully dependent on phosphatidylinositol 3-kinase-mediated signaling, is partially inhibited by rapamycin, and is independent of S6K1 and rpS6 phosphorylation. Mol Cell Biol 24: 8671–8683
11. Oldham S, Montagne J, Radimerski T, Thomas G, Hafen E (2000) Genetic and biochemical characterization of dTOR, the Drosophila homolog of the target of rapamycin. Genes Dev 14: 2689–2694
12. Zhang H, Stallock JP, Ng JC, Reinhard C, Neufeld TP (2000) Regulation of cellular growth by the Drosophila target of rapamycin dTOR. Genes Dev 14: 2712–2724
13. Montagne J, Stewart MJ, Stocker H, Hafen E, Kozma SC, Thomas G (1999) Drosophila S6 kinase: a regulator of cell size. Science 285: 2126–2129
14. Avruch J (2003) Regulation of cell growth and proliferation in metazoans by mTOR and p70S6 kinase. In: Bradshaw R and Dennis E (eds) Handbook of Cell Signaling. Chapter 87 1: 523–534
15. Hara K, Yonezawa K, Weng QP, Kozlowski MT, Belham C, Avruch J (1998) Amino acid sufficiency and mTOR regulate p70 S6 kinase and eIF-4E BP1 through a common effector mechanism. J Biol Chem 273: 14484–14494
16. Shigemitsu K, Tsujishita Y, Miyake H, Hidayat S, Tanaka N, Hara K, Yonezawa K (1999) Structural requirement of leucine for activation of p70 S6 kinase. FEBS Lett 447: 303–306
17. Xu G, Kwon G, Cruz WS, Marshall CA, McDaniel ML (2001) Metabolic regulation by leucine of translation initiation through the mTOR-signaling pathway by pancreatic beta-cells. Diabetes 50: 353–360
18. Hardie DG, Carling D, Carlson M (1998) The AMP-activated/SNF1 protein kinase subfamily: metabolic sensors of the eukaryotic cell? Annu Rev Biochem 67: 821–855

19. Kemp BE, Mitchelhill KI, Stapleton D, Michell BJ, Chen ZP, Witters LA (1999) Dealing with energy demand: the AMP-activated protein kinase. Trends Biochem Sci 24: 22–25
20. Kimura N, Tokunaga C, Dalal S, Richardson C, Yoshino K, Hara K, Kemp BE, Witters LA, Mimura O, Yonezawa K (2003) A possible linkage between AMP-activated protein kinase (AMPK) and mammalian target of rapamycin (mTOR) signaling pathway. Genes Cells 8: 65–79
21. Hara K, Maruki Y, Long X, Yoshino K, Oshiro N, Hidayat S, Tokunaga C, Avruch J, Yonezawa K (2002) Raptor, a binding partner of target of rapamycin (TOR), mediates TOR action. Cell 110: 177–189
22. Kim DH, Sarbassov DD, Ali SM, King JE, Latek RR, Erdjument-Bromage H, Tempst P, Sabatini DM (2002) mTOR interacts with raptor to form a nutrient-sensitive complex that signals to the cell growth machinery. Cell 110: 163–175
23. Loewith R, Jacinto E, Wullschleger S, Lorberg A, Crespo JL, Bonenfant D, Oppliger W, Jenoe P, Hall MN (2002) Two TOR complexes, only one of which is rapamycin sensitive, have distinct roles in cell growth control. Mol Cell 10: 457–468
24. Kim DH, Sarbassov DD, Ali SM, Latek RR, Guntur KV, Erdjument-Bromage H, Tempst P, Sabatini DM (2003) GbetaL, a positive regulator of the rapamycin-sensitive pathway required for the nutrient-sensitive interaction between raptor and mTOR. Mol Cell 11: 895–904
25. Schalm SS, Blenis J (2002) Identification of a conserved motif required for mTOR signaling. Curr Biol 12: 632–639
26. Nojima H, Tokunaga C, Eguchi S, Oshiro N, Hidayat S, Yoshino K, Hara K, Tanaka N, Avruch J, Yonezawa K (2003) The mammalian target of rapamycin (mTOR) partner, raptor, binds the mTOR substrates p70 S6 kinase and 4E-BP1 through their TOR signaling (TOS) motif. J Biol Chem 278: 15461–15464
27. Schalm SS, Fingar DC, Sabatini DM, Blenis J (2003) TOS motif-mediated raptor binding regulates 4E-BP1 multisite phosphorylation and function. Curr Biol 13: 797–806
28. Choi KM, McMahon LP, Lawrence JJ (2003) Two motifs in the translational repressor PHAS-I required for efficient phosphorylation by mammalian target of rapamycin and for recognition by raptor. J Biol Chem 278: 19667–19673
29. Beugnet A, Wang X, Proud CG (2003) Target of rapamycin (TOR)-signaling and RAIP motifs play distinct roles in the mammalian TOR-dependent phosphorylation of initiation factor 4E-binding protein 1. J Biol Chem 278: 40717–40722
30. Oshiro N, Yoshino K, Hidayat S, Tokunaga C, Hara K, Eguchi S, Avruch J, Yonezawa K (2004) Dissociation of raptor from mTOR is a mechanism of rapamycin-induced inhibition of mTOR function. Genes Cells 4: 359–366
31. Liu Z, Sekito T, Epstein CB, Butow RA (2001) RTG-dependent mitochondria to nucleus signaling is negatively regulated by the seven WD-repeat protein Lst8p. EMBO J 20: 7209–7219
32. Kwiatkowski DJ (2003) Tuberous sclerosis: from tubers to mTOR. Ann Hum Genet 67: 87–96
33. Oldham S, Hafen E (2003) Insulin/IGF and target of rapamycin signaling: a TOR de force in growth control. Trends Cell Biol 13: 79–85
34. Shamji AF, Nghiem P, Schreiber SL (2003) Integration of growth factor and nutrient signaling: implications for cancer. Mol Cell 12: 271–280
35. Manning BD, Tee AR, Logsdon MN, Blenis J, Cantley LC (2002) Identification of the tuberous sclerosis complex-2 tumor suppressor gene product tuberin as a target of the phosphoinositide 3-kinase/akt pathway. Mol Cell 10: 151–162
36. Potter CJ, Pedraza LG, Xu T (2002) Akt regulates growth by directly phosphorylating Tsc2. Nat Cell Biol 4: 658–665
37. Inoki K, Li Y, Zhu T, Wu J, Guan KL (2002) TSC2 is phosphorylated and inhibited by Akt and suppresses mTOR signalling. Nat Cell Biol 4: 648–657

38. Inoki K, Li Y, Xu T, Guan KL (2003) Rheb GTPase is a direct target of TSC2 GAP activity and regulates mTOR signaling. Genes Dev 17: 1829–1834
39. Gao X, Zhang Y, Arrazola P, Hino O, Kobayashi T, Yeung RS, Ru B, Pan D (2002) Tsc tumour suppressor proteins antagonize amino-acid-TOR signalling. Nat Cell Biol 4: 699–704
40. Saucedo LJ, Gao X, Chiarelli DA, Li L PD, Edgar BA (2003) Rheb promotes cell growth as a component of the insulin/TOR signalling network. Nat Cell Biol 5: 566–571
41. Zhang Y, Gao X, Saucedo LJ, Ru B, Edgar BA, Pan D (2003) Rheb is a direct target of the tuberous sclerosis tumour suppressor proteins. Nat Cell Biol 5: 578–581
42. Stocker H, Radimerski T, Schindelholz B, Wittwer F, Belawat P, Daram P, Breuer S, Thomas G, Hafen E (2003) Rheb is an essential regulator of S6K in controlling cell growth in Drosophila. Nat Cell Biol 5: 559–566
43. Patel PH, Thapar N, Guo L, Martinez M, Maris J, Gau CL, Lengyel JA, Tamanoi F (2003) Drosophila Rheb GTPase is required for cell cycle progression and cell growth. J Cell Sci 116: 3601–3610
44. Garami A, Zwartkruis FZT, Nobukuni T, Joaquin M, Roccio M, Stocker H, Kozma SC, Hafen E, Bos JL, Thomas G (2003) Insulin activation of Rheb, a mediator of mTOR/S6K/4E-BP signaling, is inhibited by TSC1 and 2. Mol Cell 11: 1457–1466
45. Castro AF, Rebhun JF, Clark GJ, Quilliam LA (2003) Rheb binds tuberous sclerosis complex 2 (TSC2) and promotes S6 kinase in a rapamycin- and farnesylation-dependent manner. J Biol Chem 278: 32493–32496
46. Tee A, Manning B, Roux P, Cantley L, Blenis J (2003) Tuberous sclerosis complex gene products, Tuberin and Hamartin, control mTOR signaling by acting as a GTPase-activating protein complex toward Rheb. Curr Biol 13: 1259–1268

Effect of Oral Supplementation with Branched-Chain Amino Acids on Albumin Concentration in the Early Stage of Cirrhosis

Shuhei Nishiguchi[1], Daiki Habu[1], and Susumu Shiomi[2]

Summary. The present study was undertaken to examine changes in the levels of amino acids, particularly branched-chain amino acids (BCAAs), following exacerbation of liver cirrhosis and to determine the optimal timing of starting nutritional therapy using BCAA. In patients with well-compensated cirrhosis, both the amino-acid composition and the albumin level were normal. However, as the disease advanced, BCAA first began to decrease, causing amino-acid imbalance, and this change was later followed by a decrease in albumin. We reviewed the criteria for determining indications for treatment with a BCAA formula (Livact), which is currently used after a decrease in albumin level. In patients in whom the BCAA-to-tyrosine ratio (BTR) was less than 4.0 despite normal albumin levels, the use of the BCAA preparation prevented a decrease in albumin. In view of this result, it is advisable to administer the BCAA formula following a reduction in BTR rather than to begin its use following a decrease in albumin.

Key words. Albumin, Branched-chain amino acid, Liver cirrhosis, Nutritional therapy

Introduction

Viral liver cirrhosis is sometimes treated, with agents such as interferon (IFN) and lamivudine which are related to the cause of the cirrhosis. However, many patients with this condition receive liver-protective therapy with ursodeoxycholic acid (UDCA) or other drugs that is aimed at reducing the alanine aminotransferase (ALT) level; drugs used are ursodeoxy-cholic acid (UDCA) or other drugs. The survival rate of patients with liver cirrhosis has been improved by such liver-protective therapy, by the treatment of esophageal varices, and by various other treatments. As the survival time of such patients becomes longer, the importance of diet therapy increases.

Serum albumin concentrations, which are considered to be a good and stable indicator of visceral protein nutritional status, are often low in patients with liver cirrho-

[1]Department of Hepatology, Graduate School of Medicine, Osaka City University Medical School, 1-4-3 Asahimachi, Abeno-ku, Osaka 545-8585, Japan
[2]Department of Nuclear Medicine, Graduate School of Medicine, Osaka City University, 1-4-3 Asahimachi, Abeno-ku, Osaka 545-8585, Japan

sis. This is caused not only by insufficient protein intake but also by various other factors, including reduced liver protein synthesis, increased extravascular leakage. In patients with low albumin concentration, half-life of albumin was extended to keep its level. Therefore, it is very difficult to assess serum albumin concentrations in patients with liver cirrhosis. However, it has been demonstrated that this concentration plays an important role in the prognosis of these patients [1–3]. It has been reported that prognosis generally differs between patients with a serum albumin concentration of more than 3.5 g/dl and patients with a serum albumin concentration of 3.5 g/dl or less [1]. This value (3.5 g/dl) is also used in the criteria for Child-Pugh classifications. A decrease in Fischer's ratio, i.e., the branched-chain amino acid/ aromatic amino acid (BCAA/ AAA) ratio, is an indicator of disorders of amino-acid metabolism which are characteristic of liver cirrhosis [4]. It has been reported that a decreased Fischer's ratio is not only a direct risk factor for hepatic encephalopathy (which is a significant complication of liver cirrhosis) but is also an independent prognostic factor [5].

The correction of hypoalbuminemia and the decreased Fischer's ratio, factors which closely interact and are representative indicators of malnutrition in patients with liver cirrhosis, leads to amelioration of the pathophysiological condition and prevention of deterioration in quality of life, and finally improvement of mortality rates. For these purposes, in Japan, supplementation with BCAAs is mainly used as nutritional therapy and nutritional intervention. Evidence about the usefulness of this therapy is being accumulated. In this article, among various issues relating to supplementation with BCAAs, we focus on its usefulness for patients with early-stage liver cirrhosis, which we have previously advocated.

The Purpose of BCAA Administration

A gradual decrease in the BCAA/AAA ratio is associated with the progression of chronic liver disorders [6]. Since AAAs undergo metabolism exclusively in the liver, AAA levels increase in patients with liver cirrhosis, who have decreased metabolic function [7]. It has been reported that, after liver transplantation, AAA levels rapidly return to normal as liver function recovers [8]. We have previously mentioned that portosystemic shunt causes AAAs to 'pass through' the liver, and that this may play a role in the mechanism of the increase in AAA levels in cirrhosis with Child-Pugh A [9].

On the other hand, there are various opinions about the mechanism of decreasing BCAA levels. It has been reported that hyperinsulinemia increases BCAA uptake [10], that BCAAs are increasingly consumed as energy substrates which are directly used [11], and that the consumption of BCAAs increases in accordance with increased ammonia metabolism in skeletal muscles [12]. As a result, the Fischer's ratio (BCAA/AAA) decreases, which directly and indirectly decreases serum proteins such as albumin, and destroys muscle proteins.

Originally, the purpose of using BCAA administration for the correction of Fischer's ratio focused on the awakening from hepatic encephalopathy [13]. Decreased BCAA concentrations reflect metabolic kinetics, mainly involving protein hypercatabolism. 15 years ago, Yoshida et al. [14] more than 10 years ago, started using BCAAs and showed that this therapy gave patients with liver cirrhosis an improved quality of life and an extended prognosis. Subsequently, BCAA preparations were placed on the market, and their usefulness is becoming commonly recognized. An extensive multicenter post-marketing survey of BCAA granules has recently been conducted in more than 600 patients with liver cirrhosis, and the usefulness of these granules has been confirmed. When the results of this survey are reported, they will show conclusive evidence that the administration of BCAAs to patients with liver cirrhosis not only ameliorates hepatic encephalopathy and the pathophysiological condition but also extends the prognosis of these patients by enhancing the function and reserve capacity of the liver.

Target Patients for BCAA Administration

Currently, the main target patients for nutritional therapy for liver cirrhosis are patients in the decompensated stage, who clearly exhibit clinical symptoms. The effects of treatments for peritoneal effusion and hepatic encephalopathy are easy to recognize due to the evident deterioration and resolution of these symptoms. Additionally, it only takes a short time to assess the prognosis of patients in the decompensated stage. However, there is an opinion that, for patients with liver cirrhosis, it may be better to start nutritional therapy in the compensatory stage or even earlier, rather than starting it in the decompensated stage.

We performed supplementation with BCAAs in patients in the compensatory stage of liver cirrhosis [15]. During this treatment, as an indicator of disorders of amino-acid metabolism, we used the BCAA/tyrosine ratio (BTR) instead of Fischer's ratio. The measurement method for BTR is simple and inexpensive, and BTR can generally be a substitute for Fischer's ratio, and is being commonly used in Japan [16]. The BTR of healthy people is considered to be 5.82–8.64 (mean ± 1 SD) or 4.41–10.05 (mean ± 2 SD). It has been demonstrated that BTR regularly and gradually decreases as liver diseases progress. We used platelet counts to classify 448 patients with hepatitis C virus (HCV)-related chronic liver diseases, who were outpatients at our hospital, and analyzed the mean BTR in each class ification group (Fig. 1). To obtain better correction of disorders of amino-acid metabolism and protein metabolism—which are associated with chronic liver diseases—the optimal timing of nutritional interventions with appropriate amounts of BCAA supplementation is an interesting issue.

After conducting the study with the 448 patients noted above, we studied 84 patients with Child-Pugh A liver cirrhosis in the compensatory stage, who were enrolled from March 1996 to July 1997. These patients were divided into two groups (the BTR ≥ 4 group $n = 57$ and the BTR < 4 group; $n = 27$), and were followed for up to 4 years. The percentage of these patients in whom the cirrhosis severity changed to Child-Pugh B, even transiently, was 21% in the BTR ≥ 4 group, which was significantly lower than that in the BTR < 4 group (70%). Additionally, multivariate analysis revealed that BTR was an independent risk factor for a change in the severity from Child-Pugh A to Child-Pugh B. Therefore, we considered a patient with a BTR value less than 4 as a patient with amino-acid imbalance even in the compensatory stage of liver cirrhosis, and we conducted the randomized study, outlined below, in order to make a comparison

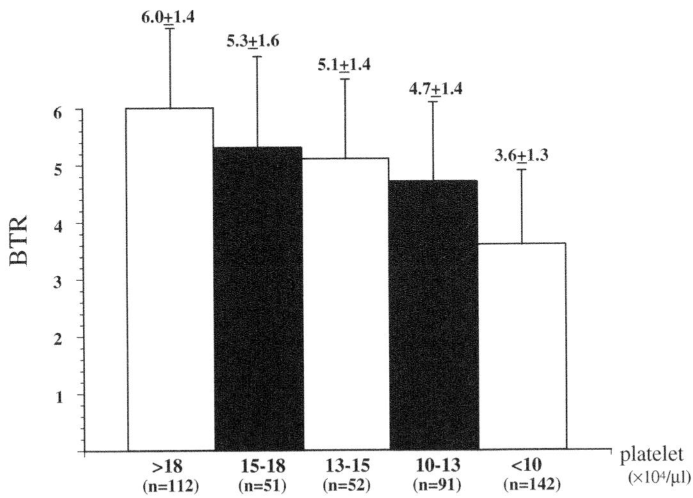

Fig. 1. The mean branched-chain amino acid (BCAA)/tyrosine ratio (*BTR*) of patients with hepatitis C virus (HCV)-related chronic liver diseases ($n = 448$), who were classified using platelet counts (mean ± SD). We used platelet counts to classify 448 patients with HCV-related chronic liver diseases, who were outpatients at our hospital, and analyzed the mean BTR in each class ification group. The BTR of healthy people is considered to be 5.82–8.64 (mean ± 1 SD) or 4.41–10.05 (mean ± 2 SD). It has been demonstrated that BTR regularly and gradually decreases as liver diseases progress.

between the effects of BCAA granules in patients who met the criterion of having a BTR value of 4 or less and patients who met the conventional criterion of having a serum albumin concentration of 3.5 g/dl or less [17]. All the subjects of this study were patients with HCV-related liver cirrhosis, and they were classified into three classes. Class 1 had a serum albumin concentration of 3.5 g/dl or less (25 patients, conventional targets of BCAA supplementation), class 2 had a serum albumin concentration between 3.6 g/dl and 3.9 g/dl and a BTR of less than 4 (18 patients), and class 3 (17 patients) had a serum albumin concentration between 3.6 g/dl and 3.9 g/dl, and a BTR of 4 or more. These patients ($n = 60$) were randomly allocated to two groups: the group that was given a BCAA preparation (Livact; Ajinomoto, Tokyo, Japan; BCAA group) and the group that was not (control group). The effect of BCAA administration was evaluated according to changes in the serum albumin concentration after 2 years as an indicator. The BCAA administration was considered to have been effective when the albumin concentration increased by 0.2 g/dl or more. The characteristics of the patients in each class are shown in Table 1. The patients continued to consume a diet that had a total daily calorie intake of 30 kcal/kg and a protein intake of 1.3 g/kg (including amino-acid preparations). The results of this study were: (1) in class 1, the effective rate (increase in serum albumin concentration of 0.2 g/dl or more) in the BCAA group was 46%, which was significantly higher than the 8% rate in the control group, (2) in class 2, the effective rate in the BCAA group was 44%, which was significantly higher than the 0% rate in the control group, and (3) in class 3, the effective rate in the BCAA group was 67%, which was not significantly different from the 36% rate in the control group (Fig. 2).

Table 1. Baseline characteristics of three classes of patients

	Class 1 (Alb ≤ 3.5)	Class 2 (Alb > 3.5; BTR < 4)	Class 3 (Alb > 3.5; BTR ≥ 4)	
Sex (male/female)	11/14	6/12	5/12	NS
BCAA/Control	13/12	9/9	6/11	NS
Average age (years)	64.3 ± 4.9	63.8 ± 7.0	67.5 ± 8.8	NS
Average BTR	3.1 ± 0.2	3.4 ± 0.5**	4.6 ± 0.3**	$P < 0.001$
Albumin (g/dl)	3.3 ± 0.2	3.8 ± 0.1**	3.8 ± 0.1**	$P < 0.001$
Platelets ($\times 10^4$/mm^3)	8.6 ± 4.8	10.4 ± 3.9*	15.1 ± 5.8*	$P < 0.01$
ALT (IU/l)	117.0 ± 84.0	98.4 ± 42.7	79.4 ± 38.1	NS
Bilirubin (mg/dl)	1.3 ± 0.5	1.0 ± 0.3	0.9 ± 0.4	NS

Wilcoxon rank-sum test for age, BTR (branched-chain amino-acid (BCAA)/tyrosine ratio), serum albumin, platelets, alanine aminotransferase (ALT), and total bilirubin; χ^2 test for sex ratio and BCAA/control ratio (adapted from reference [23])

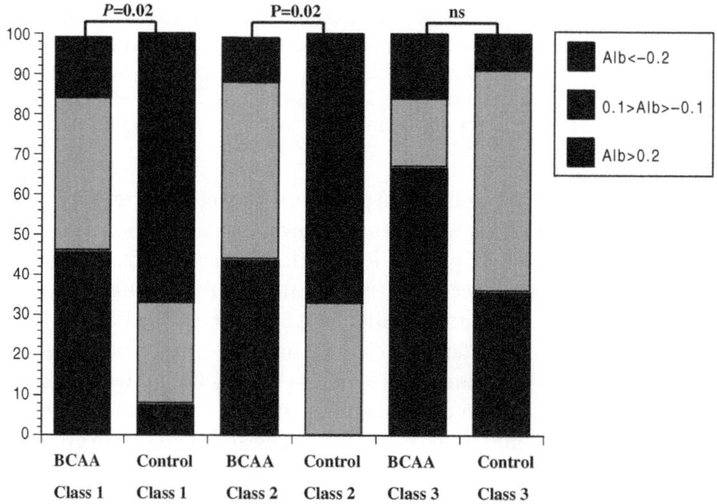

Fig. 2. Comparison of serum albumin (*alb*) levels at 2 years after study enrollment between the BCAA and control groups in class 1, class 2, and class 3. Patients in class 1 had decompensated cirrhosis, with a serum albumin concentration of 3.5 g/dl or less. Class 2 patients had compensated cirrhosis, with a serum albumin concentration between 3.6 g/dl and 3.9 g/dl, and a BTR of less than 4. Class 3 patients had compensated cirrhosis, with a serum albumin concentration between 3.6 g/dl and 3.9 g/dl, and a BTR of 4 or more. The BCAA groups in classes 1 and 2 exhibited a significantly higher rate of maintaining serum albumin levels compared with that at enrollment in the respective control groups (χ^2 test for independence, $P = 0.02$), but the difference between the BCAA group and the control group in class 3 was not significant (*ns*). (adapted from reference [17])

Table 2. Odds ratios for decrease in serum albumin level 2 years after study enrollment in the control group

	Odds ratio	95% CI	*P* Value
Serum albumin	1.586	0.281–8.960	0.6015
BTR	9.444	1.524–58.521	0.0158
Total bilirubin	0.463	0.071–3.028	0.4214
ALT	1.549	0.322–7.452	0.5849
Platelet count	5.619	0.954–33.101	0.0564

Odds ratios for risk factors are expressed as per 1 year for age. The values for all parameters in Table 4 were each categorized into two groups: albumin, >3.5 and ≤3.5 g/dl; BTR, ≥4.0 and <4; total bilirubin, ≤1.0 and >1.0; ALT level, <80 and ≥80 IU/ml; platelet count, ≥100 000 and <100 000/mm^3, and odds ratios are indicated for each set of two groups (adapted from reference [17])
CI, confidence interval

Additionally, in the control group, which was followed up without BCAA administration, we performed multivariate analysis to determine the defining factors in the decrease in serum albumin concentrations 2 years after study enrollment, and found that BTR was the only risk factor (Table 2). The results of this study showed that, in patients with liver cirrhosis in the compensatory stage classified in class 2 who had relatively constant serum albumin concentrations (between 3.6 g/dl and 3.9 g/dl), when amino-acid imbalance was manifested (BTR < 4), the administration of BCAA granules increased the serum albumin concentrations to levels similar to those observed in the patients in the decompensated stage.

We assume that when BCAA therapy is not given to patients in class 2, the decreased Fischer's ratio will trigger a decrease in albumin synthesis, and their condition is likely to progress to Child-Pugh B (serum albumin, 3.5 g/dl or less). Consequently, we assume that, in many patients with liver cirrhosis, as the compensatory stage progresses, the Fischer's ratio decreases prior to a decrease in serum albumin concentration (Fig. 3).

The mechanism whereby BCAA administration increases serum albumin concentration is shown in detail in the chapter by K. Yonezawa. It has been assumed that the correction of Fischer's ratio promotes protein synthesis [18], improves the metabolic kinetics of albumin [19], and inhibits proteolysis [20]. Therefore, in patients in the conpensatory stage with high serum albumin levels, low BTR level or low Fisher's ratio in the correction of Fischer's ratio by BCAA administration may prevent a decrease in albumin synthesis.

It has been demonstrated that when patients with advanced liver cirrhosis are given BCAA granules, serum albumin concentrations do not increase sufficiently, because these patients have only a small total number of functioning hepatocytes. At present, it is assumed that only such cells (liver parenchymal cells) can synthesize albumin. Therefore, the results of this study suggest that the administration of BCAA granules is more effective in increasing and maintaining serum albumin concentrations when it is started at an early stage, of patients who have a sufficient number of functioning hepatocytes (the total number of cells which can synthesize albumin by BCAA).

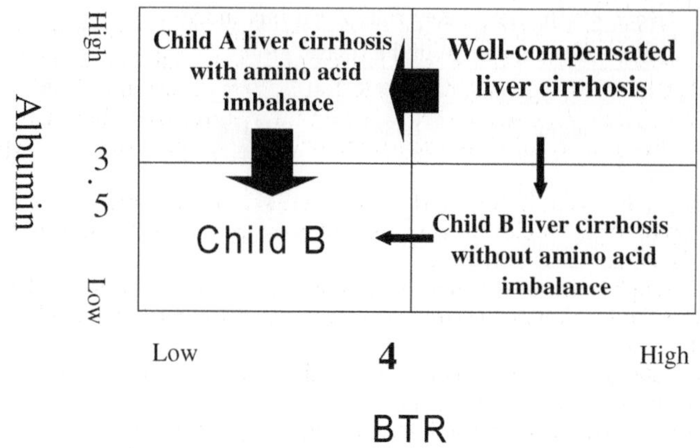

Fig. 3. Progression of compensated liver cirrhosis to decompensated liver cirrhosis. It is assumed that, in the majority of patients during the progression of compensated liver cirrhosis, Fischer's ratio decreases (*large arrows*) prior to a decrease in serum albumin concentration.

References

1. Zoli M, Cordiani MR, Marchesini G, Iervese T, Labate AM, Bonazzi C, Bianchi G (1991) Prognostic indicators in compensated cirrhosis. Am J Gastroenterol 86: 1508–1513
2. Guechot J, Serfaty L, Bonnand AM, Chazouilleres O, Poupon RE, Poupon R (2000) Prognostic value of serum hyaluronan in patients with compensated HCV cirrhosis. J Hepatol 32: 447–452
3. Luo JC, Hwang SJ, Chang FY, Chu CW, Lai CR, Wang YJ, Lee PC, Tsay SH, Lee SD (2002) Simple blood tests can predict compensated liver cirrhosis in patients with chronic hepatitis C. Hepatogastroenterology 49: 478–481
4. Rosen HM, Yoshimura N, Hodgman JM, Fischer JE (1977) Plasma amino acid pattern in hepatic encephalopathy of different etiology. Gastroenterology 72: 483–487
5. Tajika M, Kato M, Mohri H, Miwa Y, Kato T, Ohnishi H, Moriwaki H (2002) Prognostic value of energy metabolism in patients with viral liver cirrhosis. Nutrition 18: 229–234
6. Morgan MY, Milsom JP, Sherlock S (1978) Plasma ratio of valine, leucine and isoleucine to phenylalanine and tyrosine in liver disease. Gut 19: 1068–1073
7. O'Keefe SJD, Abraham R, EL-Zayadi A, Marshall W, Davis M, Williams R (1981) Increased plasma tyrosine concentrations in patients with cirrhosis and fulminant hepatic failure associated with increased plasma tyrosine flux and related hepatic oxidation capacity. Gastroenterology 81: 1017–1024
8. Tietge UFJ, Bahr MJ, Manns MP, Boker KH (2002) Plasma amino acids in cirrhosis and after liver transplantation: influence of liver function, hepatic hemodynamics and circulating hormones. Clin Transplant 16: 9–17
9. Habu D, Nishiguchi S, Nakatani S, Kawamura E, Ishizu H, Lee C, Ohfuji S, Fukushima W, Tanaka T, Kawamura T, Shiomi S (2003) Relationship between branched-chain amino acid to tyrosine ratio (BTR) and porto-systemic shunt in the early stage of cirrhosis determined by per-rectal portal scintigraphy. Hepatol Res 27: 57–61
10. Marchesini G, Forlani G, Zoli M, Dondi C, Bianchi G, Bua V, Vannini P, Pisi E (1983) Effect of euglycemic insulin infusion on plasma levels of branched-chain amino acids in cirrhosis. Hepatology 3: 184–187

11. Wannemacher RW Jr. (1977) Key role of various individual amino acids in host response to infection. Am J Clin Nutr 30: 1269–1280
12. Hayashi M, Ohnishi H, KawadaY, Muto Y, Takanashi Y (1981) Augmented utilization of branched-chain amino acids by skeletal muscle in decompensated liver cirrhosis in special relation to ammonia detoxication. Gastroenterol Jpn 64: 64–70
13. Fabbri A, Magrini N, Bianchi G, Zoli M, Marchesini G (1996) Overview of randomized clinical trials of oral branched-chain amino acid treatment in chronic hepatic encephalopathy. J Parenter Enteral Nutr 20: 159–164
14. Yoshida T, Muto Y, Moriwaki H, Yamato M (1989) Effect of long-term oral supplementation with branched-chain amino acid granules on the prognosis of liver cirrhosis. Gastroenterol Jpn 24: 692–698
15. Habu D, Nishiguchi S, Nakatani N, Kawamura E, Lee C, Enomoto M, Tamori A, Takeda T, Tanaka T, Shiomi S (2003) Effect of oral supplementation with branched-chain amino acid granules on serum albumin level in the early stage of cirrhosis: a randomized pilot study. Hepatol Res 25: 312–318
16. Azuma Y, Maekawa M, Kuwabara Y, Nakajima T, Taniguchi K, Kanno T (1989) Determination of branched-chain amino acids and tyrosine in serum of patients with various hepatic diseases, and its clinical usefulness. Clin Chem 35: 1399–1403
17. Habu D, Nishiguchi S, Nakatani S, Kawamura E, Lee C, Enomoto M, Tamori A, Takeda T, Tanaka T, Shiomi S. Comparison of the effect of oral supplementation with branched-chain amino acid on serum albumin level between decompensated cirrhosis and compensated cirrhosis. Hepatogastroenterology
18. Okuno M, Moriwaki H, Kato M, Muto Y, Kojima S (1995) Changes in the ratio of branched-chain to aromatic amino acids affect the secretion of albumin in cultured rat hepatocytes. Biochem Biophys Res Commun 214: 1045–1050
19. Usui T, Moriwaki H, Hatakeyama H, Kasai T, Kato M, Seishima M, Okuno M, Ohnishi H, Yoshida T, Muto Y (1996) Oral supplementation with branched-chain amino acids improves transthyretin turnover in rats with carbon tetrachloride-induced liver cirrhosis. J Nutr 126: 1412–1420
20. Marchesini G, Zoli M, Dondi C, Bianchi G, Cirulli M, Pisi E (1982) Anticatabolic effect of branched-chain amino acid-enriched solutions in patients with liver cirrhosis. Hepatology 2: 420–425

Nutritional Therapy in Patients with Liver Cirrhosis

Masako Tsuchiya, Isao Sakaida, Mariko Okamoto, and Kiwamu Okita

Summary. As an intervention for energy malnutrition in patients with liver cirrhosis, frequent meals or a late evening snack (LES) have recently been recommended. We investigated which would be better for the improvement of energy malnutrition and glucose intolerance in cirrhotic patients, treatment with an LES alone or an LES plus divided meals. We examined one group of cirrhotic patients that received oral supplementation with one pack of a branched-chain amino acid (BCAA)-enriched nutrient, Aminoleban EN (210 Kcal), taken at 10 p.m. as an LES, and a second group that received two packs of Aminoleban EN (one pack as an LES, and one pack taken during the day) to determine the influence of the LES on the blood glucose level, biochemical parameters, and energy metabolism. The administration period was 7 days. Metabolic measurements were performed using indirect calorimetry. The fat oxidation rate was significantly decreased and the carbohydrate oxidation rate was significantly increased in both groups. As a result, the respiratory quotient (RQ) was significantly improved. There was also a significant correlation between the nonprotein respiratory quotient (npRQ) and the creatinine-height index. LES alone improved the energy malnutrition state and glucose intolerance equivalent to LES plus divided meals.

Key words. Liver cirrhosis, Nutrition, Glucose intolerance, LES, OGTT

Introduction

Liver diseases lead to abnormalities in nutrient metabolism and subsequent malnutrition [1]. Protein-energy malnutrition (PEM) is a common finding in cirrhotic patients [2–5]. Owen et al. [6] reported that, after an overnight fast, the nature of fuels oxidized in cirrhotic patients was similar to that in healthy controls after 2 to 3 days of total starvation; that is, there was a relatively high contribution of fat to energy metabolism. Several studies have reported that the protein nutrition state and malnutrition determine the survival rate of cirrhotic patients [7]. Nutritional support for protein malnutrition partly improves the survival rate and surgical outcome of these

Department of Gastroenterology and Hepatology, Yamaguchi University School of Medicine, 1-1-1 Minami-Kogushi, Ube, Yamaguchi 755-8505, Japan patients [3, 4, 8–11], although there have been some criticisms of the hypothesis of the nutritional state as a survival factor or therapeutic strategy [12, 13].

Therefore, special attention is required in the management of these patients. Proper nutritional assessment and support for cirrhotic patients is very important. As an intervention for energy malnutrition, either frequent meals or a late evening snack (LES) have recently been recommended [14–18]. In liver cirrhosis, the supply of glucose from the liver is disturbed and, thus, energy utilization from lipids and proteins is accelerated [19]. Furthermore, excess elevation of blood glucose occurs after meals in liver cirrhosis. It has been reported that glucose intolerance is found in approximately 70% of patients with liver cirrhosis, and in about 40% of those with diabetes [20, 21]. Bianchi et al. [22] reported that diabetes affected the survival rate in patients with cirrhosis. In this study, we examined the effects of LES alone and LES plus divided meals on the metabolism, using indirect calorimetry and the changes in blood glucose levels after meals.

Subjects and Methods

This study was performed in 20 patients with liver cirrhosis hospitalized in our hospital. The patients, aged from 45 to 77 years, consisted of 12 men and 8 women. Liver cirrhosis was caused by hepatitis B virus (HBV) in 1 patient and by HCV in 19 patients.

We investigated the effect of nutrition in two groups, one group that received oral supplementation of one pack of Aminoleban EN at 10 p.m. as an LES, and another group that received two packs of Aminoleban EN, one taken at 10 p.m. as an LES, and the other taken during the daytime (the period from 10 a.m. to 3 p.m.). Aminoleban EN is an oral supplement enriched with branched-chain amino acids (BCAAs) and is comprised mainly of carbohydrate (59%), protein (26%), and fat (15%), which allows a high protein intake.

Energy metabolism at baseline was analyzed by indirect calorimetry. Indirect calorimetry was performed for 30 min after overnight bedrest and fasting. The indirect calorimeter used was a calorie scale (Chest, MI, USA). We measured oxygen consumption per min (VO_2), carbon dioxide production per min (VCO_2), and total urine nitrogen (TUN) on the day prior to the examination, and fat oxidation and the nonprotein respiratory quotient (npRQ) were calculated. Calculation of the diet for each patient was based on the following conditions: 30–35 kcal/kg per day as total calories for ideal body weight (body mass index [BMI], 22), with 1–1.5 g protein/kg per day and fat content equivalent to 25% of the total calories. During LES administration, reduced-calorie diets were used, i.e., calories equivalent to the amounts in two packs or one pack of Aminoleban EN (210 kcal/pack; protein, 13.5 g/pack; fat, 3.5 g/pack) were subtracted. The administration period was 7 days; the calorie consumption of all patients was checked by a nutrition technician and all patients took the prescribed calorie content. On days 1 and 7, we performed nutritional evaluation, by indirect calorimetry, and we determined the blood glucose level, and carried out biochemical examinations. Changes in the blood glucose level were measured at seven time points: 30 min before and 2 h after each meal and at 10 p.m. The levels before meals and those after meals on days 1 and 7 were compared. The BCAA/tyrosine ratio

(BTR) [23] was also examined on days 1 and 7. The BTR is the molar ratio of (valine + leucine + isoleucine)/tyrosine, determined by measuring only tyrosine as an aromatic amino acid (AAA), and it is different from the Fischer ratio. Besides indirect calorimetry, nutrition evaluation was based on the biochemical parameters, serum albumin, and anthropometric parameters, i.e., BMI and the creatinine-height index (CHI).

Statistical Analysis

Data values were expressed as means ± SE. Two-tailed *t*-tests were used to compare means for continuous variables. Nonparametric methods were also used for nonnormally distributed values, and differences were tested by the Wilcoxon signed rank test. To calculate correlation coefficients between selected variables, the Spearman rank correlation coefficient was used. For all tests, P values of less than 0.05 were considered significant.

Results

Indirect Calorimetry

The npRQ value in both groups increased significantly after 1-week treatment (one-pack group; baseline, 0.82 ± 0.03 vs 0.88 ± 0.03; $P < 0.05$; two-pack group; baseline, 0.76 ± 0.03 vs 0.81 ± 0.02; $P < 0.05$). The fat oxidation rate as an energy substrate decreased significantly with an increase in the glucose oxidation rate.

BTR Measurement

A significant increase in BTR was also observed after treatment (one-pack group, baseline, 3.10 ± 1.01 vs 4.41 ± 1.01; $P < 0.05$; two-pack group, baseline, 3.60 ± 1.45 vs 5.25 ± 2.01; $P < 0.05$). However, no significant difference was observed in the blood ammonia level (data not shown).

Changes in the Blood Glucose Level

In this study, none of the subjects had an abnormal increase in the blood glucose level before breakfast. When we checked the changes in blood glucose levels before the LES administration, five subjects had an excess increase in the blood glucose level after meals, especially after breakfast. In this study, five patients had glucose intolerance (three in the LES-alone group and two in the LES-plus-divided-meal group), with an increased blood glucose level of more than 200 mg/dl 2 h after breakfast, lunch, or dinner before the nutritional intervention. However, nutritional support for only 1 week reduced this excess increase in the glucose level after the meals, reducing it to less than 200 mg/dl (data not shown).

We investigated changes in the area under the curve (AUC) for the blood glucose level after meals before and after the nutritional support. The AUC of the one-pack group had decreased significantly (82.1 ± 13.5%; $P < 0.05$) as compared to that before the treatment (100%). Although the AUC of the two-pack group tended to decrease compared to that before the treatment, there was no significant difference (91.3 ± 20.8%). There was no significant elevation of the blood glucose level before breakfast after the 1-week treatment in either group.

Changes in npRQ According to Child-Pugh Classification

The effect of nutritional intervention on the changes in npRQ was examined in the two groups according to the Child-Pugh classification. Patients in Child-Pugh groups A and B showed an improved npRQ after the treatment, either with LES alone or LES plus divided meals ($P < 0.05$; Child-Pugh A; $n = 4$ in each group, Child-Pugh B; $n = 4$ in each group). However, for the patients who had severe decompensated cirrhosis (Child-Pugh C), nutritional treatment did not improve the npRQ ($n = 2$ in each group).

Correlation Between npRQ and Biochemical and Nutritional Parameters

We examined the correlation between npRQ and various parameters. There was a significant correlation between the value of npRQ after nutritional treatment and the CHI ($P < 0.05$), as well as a significant correlation for the change in npRQ after treatment (npRQ after treatment minus npRQ before treatment) and the CHI ($P < 0.05$), but there were no significant correlations between npRQ and BMI, albumin, total bilirubin, ammonia, or any other parameters.

Discussion

It has been reported that, after an overnight fast, the nature of fuels oxidized in cirrhotics was similar to that in healthy controls after 2 to 3 days of total starvation [24]. However, in a more recent study, Yamashita et al. [25] reported that glucose oxidation in peripheral tissue after eating was intact or increased in cirrhotics.

In the present study, we showed that LES (as in the one-pack group) and LES plus divided meals (as in the two-pack group) were very effective for morning starvation. The presence of a severe catabolic state in cirrhotic patients results in the loss of muscle, and in malnutrition, resulting in a poor prognosis [4, 7]. In both the one-pack and the two-pack groups, the npRQ improved significantly, with increased carbohydrate oxidation. The two-pack group tended to have more increased BTR than the one-pack group, but, in both groups, the value of BTR after treatment was elevated to more than 4.0. One-pack LES treatment significantly decreased the AUC, but, unexpectedly, the reductive effect on AUC with the LES plus divided meals was less than that of the LES-alone group. Other researchers have reported that the problem of glucose intolerance and diabetes in cirrhotic patients is the excess elevation of blood glucose after meals [20, 21]. In our study, before nutritional treatment, no patient had an abnormally high glucose level before breakfast, but some had an excess increase of blood glucose level after meals, especially after breakfast. Nutritional treatment reduced such elevation of the glucose level after 1 week in both groups. These results suggest that LES-alone treatment with one pack of BCAA-enriched supplement will have an effect on energy metabolism and blood glucose level equivalent to that of treatment with LES and divided meals.

Our study indicated that patients in the compensated stage, i.e., Child-Pugh A or B, will respond to the nutritional intervention easily. However, a long-term study is necessary to determine whether patients in the decompensated stage (i.e., Child-Pugh C) will respond to nutritional intervention such as the LES.

In our study, we showed that there was a significant correlation between npRQ and the creatinine-height index (CHI). The CHI is useful, as it reflects skeletal muscle volume [26]. Although the liver is considered to be the major site of amino-acid degradation [27], skeletal muscles are also another important site for amino-acid metabolism [28]. Our results suggest that muscle is also very important for the uptake and utilization of the LES nutritional supplement. That is, it is important to maintain proper muscles and, in order to do that, it is necessary to ingest suitable protein and perform appropriate exercise.

Recent studies have suggested that leucine may play an especially important role in skeletal muscles for the regulation of protein synthesis and for glucose metabolism [29–31]. This suggests that muscles may play an important role not only in amino-acid and ammonia metabolism but also in the improvement of glucose intolerance. Our results (i.e., the increase of npRQ) show that muscle volume will affect the improvement of energy metabolism, a result which coincides with these reports [29–31].

There are different opinions as to the best substrate for nutrition and the best method of administration for cirrhotic patients [32]. In cirrhotic patients, impaired glucose tolerance and insulin resistance are often observed. Nakaya et al. [33] reported that, among a BCAA mixture, a carbohydrate-rich snack (rice ball), and oral glucose with equal caloric value, oral glucose resulted in the greatest increase in the blood glucose level. Certainly, long-term oral administration of BCAA increased serum albumin in patients with cirrhosis, leading to a better quality of life (QOL) and prognosis [34]. For these reasons, we selected Aminoleban EN, a BCAA and glucose mixture also containing vitamins and trace elements that are usually lacking in patients with liver cirrhosis. However, further study is necessary to determine whether Aminoleban EN is better than a light glucose-rich snack as an LES.

In conclusion, the LES improved energy malnutrition, corrected amino-acid imbalance, and improved glucose intolerance in patients with liver cirrhosis; the effects of longer-term administration of an LES on prognosis and QOL must be investigated in the future.

References

1. Italian Multicentre Cooperative Project on Nutrition in Liver Cirrhosis. Nutritional status in cirrhosis (1994) J Hepatol 21: 317–325
2. Muller MJ (1995) Malnutrition in cirrhosis. J Hepatol 23 (Suppl 1): 31–35
3. Alberino F, Gatta A, Amodio P, et al. (2001) Nutrition and survival in patients with liver cirrhosis. Nutrition 17: 445–450
4. Tajika M, Kato M, Mohri H, et al. (2002) Prognostic value of energy metabolism in patients with viral liver cirrhosis. Nutrition 18: 229–234
5. Lautz HU, Selberg O, Korber J, et al. (1992) Protein-calorie malnutrition in liver cirrhosis. Clin Invest 70: 478–486

6. Owen OE, Trapp VE, Reichard GA Jr, et al. (1983) Nature and quantity of fuels consumed in patients with alcoholic cirrhosis. J Clin Invest 72: 1821–1832
7. O'Keefe SJ, El-Zayadi AR, Carraher TE, et al. (1980) Malnutrition and immunoincompetence in patients with liver disease. Lancet II: 615–617
8. Selberg O, Bottcher J, Tusch G, et al. (1997) Identification of high- and low-risk patients before liver transplantation: a prospective cohort study of nutritional and metabolic parameters in 150 patients. Hepatology 25: 652–657
9. Kondrup J, Muller MJ (1997) Energy and protein requirements of patients with chronic liver disease. J Hepatol 27: 239–247
10. Cabre E, Gonzalez-Huix F, Abad-Lacruz A, et al. (1990) Effect of total enteral nutrition on the short-term outcome of severely malnourished cirrhotics. A randomized controlled trial. Gastroenterology 98: 715–720
11. Hirsch S, de la Maza MP, Gattas V, et al. (1999) Nutritional support in alcoholic cirrhotic patients improves host defenses. J Am Coll Nutr 18: 434–441
12. Christie ML, Sack DM, Pomposelli J, et al. (1985) Enriched branched-chain amino acid formula versus a casein-based supplement in the treatment of cirrhosis. JPEN J Parenter Enteral Nutr 9: 671–678
13. McGhee A, Henderson JM, Millikan WJ Jr, et al. (1983) Comparison of the effects of Hepatic-Aid and a Casein modular diet on encephalopathy, plasma amino acids, and nitrogen balance in cirrhotic patients. Ann Surg 197: 288–293
14. Swart GR, Zillikens MC, van Vuure JK, et al. (1989) Effect of a late evening meal on nitrogen balance in patients with cirrhosis of the liver. BMJ 299: 1202–1203
15. Chang WK, Chao YC, Tang HS, et al. (1997) Effects of extra-carbohydrate supplementation in the late evening on energy expenditure and substrate oxidation in patients with liver cirrhosis. JPEN J Parenter Enteral Nutr 21: 96–99
16. Zillikens MC, van den Berg JW, Wattimena JL, et al. (1993) Nocturnal oral glucose supplementation. The effects on protein metabolism in cirrhotic patients and in healthy controls. J Hepatol 17: 377–383
17. Miwa Y, Shiraki M, Kato M, et al. (2000) Improvement of fuel metabolism by nocturnal energy supplementation in patients with liver cirrhosis. Hepatol Res 18: 184–189
18. Yamauchi M, Takeda K, Sakamoto K, et al. (2001) Effect of oral branched chain amino acid supplementation in the late evening on the nutritional state of patients with liver cirrhosis. Hepatol Res 21: 199–204
19. Krahenbuhl S, Reichen J (1993) Decreased hepatic glucose production in rats with carbon tetrachloride-induced cirrhosis. J Hepatol 19: 64–70
20. Muller MJ, Pirlich M, Balks HJ, et al. (1994) Glucose intolerance in liver cirrhosis: role of hepatic and non-hepatic influences. Eur J Clin Chem Clin Biochem 32: 749–758
21. Custro N, Carroccio A, Ganci A, et al. (2001) Glycemic homeostasis in chronic viral hepatitis and liver cirrhosis. Diabetes Metab 27: 476–481
22. Bianchi G, Marchesini G, Zoli M, et al. (1994) Prognostic significance of diabetes in patients with cirrhosis. Hepatology 20: 119–125
23. Kawamura-Yasui N, Kaito M, Nakagawa N, et al. (1999) Evaluating response to nutritional therapy using the branched-chain amino acid/tyrosine ratio in patients with chronic liver disease. J Clin Lab Anal 13: 31–34
24. Owen OE, Reichle FA, Mozzoli MA, et al. (1981) Hepatic, gut, and renal substrate flux rates in patients with hepatic cirrhosis. J Clin Invest 68: 240–252
25. Yamashita S, Suzuki C, Tanigawa K, et al. (1999) Glucose utilization after administration of glucose in patients with cirrhosis. Acta Hepatol Jpn 40: 636–644
26. Blackburn GL, Bistrian BR, Maini BS, et al. (1977) Nutritional and metabolic assessment of the hospitalized patient. JPEN J Parenter Enteral Nutr 1: 11–22
27. Miller LL, Holden JT (1962) The role of the liver and the non-hepatic tissues in the regulation of free amino acid levels in the blood. In: Holden JT (ed) Amino Acid Pools. Elsevier, Amsterdam, p 708

28. Kato M, Miwa Y, Tajika M, et al. (1998) Preferential use of branched-chain amino acids as an energy substrate in patients with liver cirrhosis. Intern Med 37: 429–434
29. Proud CG (2002) Regulation of mammalian translation factors by nutrients. Eur J Biochem 269: 5338–5349
30. Lynch CL (2001) Role of leucine in the regulation of mTOR by amino acids: revelations from structure-activity studies. J Nutr 131: 861S–865S
31. Anthony JC, Yoshizawa F, Anthony TG, et al. (2000) Leucine stimulates translation initiation in skeletal muscle of postabsorptive rats via a rapamycin-sensitive pathway. J Nutr 130: 2413–2419
32. Swart GR, van den Berg JW, van Vuure JK, et al. (1989) Minimum protein requirements in liver cirrhosis determined by nitrogen balance measurements at three levels of protein intake. Clin Nutr 8: 329–336
33. Nakaya Y, Harada N, Kakui S, et al. (2002) Severe catabolic state after prolonged fasting in cirrhotic patients: effect of oral branched-chain amino-acid-enriched nutrient mixture. J Gastroenterol 37: 531–536
34. Marchesini G, Bianchi G, Merli M, et al. (2003) Nutritional supplementation with branched-chain amino acids in advanced cirrhosis: a double-blind, randomized trial. Gastroenterology 124: 1792–1801

Subject Index

GPSR Compliance

The European Union's (EU) General Product Safety Regulation (GPSR) is a set of rules that requires consumer products to be safe and our obligations to ensure this.

If you have any concerns about our products, you can contact us on ProductSafety@springernature.com

In case Publisher is established outside the EU, the EU authorized representative is:

Springer Nature Customer Service Center GmbH
Europaplatz 3
69115 Heidelberg, Germany

Batch number: 10682570

Printed by Printforce, the Netherlands